ANA Workplace Health and Safety Guide for Nurses:

OSHA and NIOSH Resources

Michelle Kom Gochnour, MN, COHN-S, RN

Michelle Nawar, MA, MPH

Susan Q. Wilburn, MPH, BSN, RN

ANA
AMERICAN NURSES
ASSOCIATION

WASHINGTON, D.C.

Library of Congress Cataloging-in-Publication Data

ANA workplace health and safety guide for nurses : OSHA and NIOSH resources / by
Michelle Kom Gochnour, Michelle Nawar, and Susan Q. Wilburn
    p. ; cm.
  Includes bibliographical references.
  ISBN 1-55810-161-6
  1. Nursing–Safety measures.   I: Title: American Nurses Association workplace health and
safety guide for nurses.   II. Workplace health and safety guide for nurses.   III. Nawar, Michelle.
IV. Wilburn, Susan Q. 1955-   V. American Nurses Association.   VI. Title.
  [DNLM: 1. United States. Occupational Safety and Health Administration.   2. National
Institute for Occupational Safety and Health.   3. Health facilities–legislation & jurisprudence–
United States–Nurses' Instruction.   4. Occupational Health–legislation & jurisprudence–
United States–Nurses' Instruction.   5. Accidents, Occupational–prevention & control–United
States–Nurses' Instruction. Occupational Diseases–prevention & control–United States–Nurses'
Instruction. WA 33 AA1 G576a 2001]
RT87.S24 G63 2001
  610.73'028'9–dc21

                     2001022093

ISBN 1-55810-161-6

WPHS21   2.5M   04/01

CONTENTS

FOREWORD

Dear Colleagues,

Every day registered nurses face numerous occupational safety and health hazards, wherever they work. Technological advances plus the increasing scope of health care services and products compound these potential health threats. Historic hazards such as back injuries and exposure to bloodborne pathogens are now joined by new chemicals, vapors, and laser hazards. Well known infectious agents like TB are gaining resistance to antibiotics and therefore pose heightened risk. In addition, there are infectious agents like Hepatitis C which currently has no preventive vaccine, yet the sero-conversion rate after needle-stick injury is much higher than seen in Hepatitis B and HIV needlestick exposure.

This message is not written to increase your alarm but rather heighten your awareness of how you can reduce the potential health and safety hazards in your workplace. First, you have rights and protections under the law to help you develop a safer workplace. Read about these laws and learn the steps you can follow to address these issues.

ANA and its 54 constituent member state nurses associations work together to provide the information, guidance, tools and expertise you need in the workplace. These tools are only as effective as the individuals who make use of them. Each nurse has a responsibility to both patients and colleagues to be a part of the solution. Please make your state nurses association the first call when you need help. They also have this guidebook plus a wealth of resources that can guide you through the process.

Often, legal expertise is also needed. You need to know the laws that protect you as well as potential risks involved in reporting problems. Working with your association can help you proceed in an informed and safe manner. We look forward to working with you to make all work settings a healthy and safe place for nurses and their patients.

Sincerely,

Mary Foley, MS, RN
President
American Nurses Association

ACKNOWLEDGMENTS

The authors wish to thank the following individuals for their contribution to the development and review of the original or subsequent manuscripts for this book.

Nancey Agard, RN, former Associate Director Nursing Practice, New York State Nurses Association

Evelyn Bain, MS, RN, OHN-S, Association Director Nursing Practice, Health and Safety, Massachusetts Nurses Association

Alicia Camacho, RN, former Assoc Director E & GW Program, New York State Nurses Association

Joanne DeJanovich, MSN, RN, former Chief Executive Officer, Arkansas Nurses Association

Lisa Frascogna, JD, RN, former Health Affairs Coordinator of the Mississippi Nurses Association

Mary Griffith, MN, RNC, Director, Legislation for the Arizona Nurses Association

Kathryn V. Hall, RN, MS, Executive Director of the Maryland Nurses Association and Member

Gwen Johnson, RN, Health and Safety Officer, DC Nurses Association

Susan Johnston-Lynx, RN, JD, former program Director, Practice, Education and Policy, Minnesota Nurses Association

Clair Jordan, MSN, RN, Executive Director Texas Nurses Association

Nancy Kaleda, New York State Nurses Association

Maureen Keenan, JD, Director of Health Policy and Workplace Advocacy, Kentucky Nurses Association

Julie Pinkham, MS, RN, former Director, Labor Relations Program, Massachusetts Nurses Association

Sue Scheider, JD, Labor Representative, DC Nurses Association

Richard Schlegel, BA, Executive Director Nevada Nurses Association

Elizabeth Shogren, RN, Labor Representative, Minnesota Nurses Association

Evelyn Sommers, MBA, ED, DC Nurses Association

Betsy Waid, JD, former E & GW Program Director, Ohio Nurses Association

ANA Staff

Patty Franklin
Senior Staff Specialist
Center for Workplace Advocacy

Anna Gilmore-Hall
Director, Department of Nurse Advocacy Programs

Karen Worthington
Senior Occupational Health and Safety Specialist
Center for Occupational Safety and Health

INTRODUCTION

A Case Study: DCNA Nurses Confront Tuberculosis

Is tuberculosis a real health risk to RNs? Absolutely. If the necessary precautions are not taken, health care workers can be exposed to the highly contagious tuberculosis (TB) bacterium.

What if your hospital claims that all that you need to do is wear a surgical mask to be safe, but you know that it provides little protection? Can you do anything to change the siuation? Do you have rights or protections in place? The answer to all of these questions is a resounding "YES!" You can file a complaint with OSHA and compel your hospital to comply with the law.

At the Washington Hospital Center (WHC) in Washington, D.C., a nurse filed a complaint and OSHA came and inspected the hospital. "This case demonstrated the importance of employees taking the initiative with health and safety issues," said Sue Scheider, DCNA staff attorney.

Staff nurses provided information about the hospital's TB policies and practices. As a result, OSHA found that WHC did not use appropriate respirators. Instead, employees were instructed to wear surgical masks which do not protect them. OSHA also found that the WHC was not properly using isolation rooms. The hospital was fined and required to purchase the appropriate respirators and to construct additional isolation rooms with negative pressure capability. "It was so rewarding to see that, with an OSHA inspection, we were able to force WHC to purchase the HEPA masks [respirators] to provide a safe work environment," stated Mindy Blandon, RN.

There are federal laws that protect all workers. In 1970, after years of lobbying by the American Nurses Association (ANA) and others, Congress passed the Occupational Safety and Health (OSH) Act. The OSH Act assures "every working man and woman a safe and healthful workplace." It also established the Occupational Safety and Health Administration (OSHA), the federal agency responsible for enforcing the provisions of the OSH Act by setting safety and health standards.

This law and agency provide protection and resources for all workers, including you. Read further. This guide is both an instructional manual and a valuable reference to the laws and resources which you can use to create a healthy and safe workplace.

Using This Guide

ANA developed this guide to give nurses useful tools and knowledge to improve health and safety conditions in the workplace. The first chapter explains the legal rights and privileges extended to every worker under the Occupational Safety and Health (OSH) Act and how to execute those rights.

The second chapter focuses on how to collect and analyze data using the Occupational Safety and Health Administration (OSHA) 200 Log. Your facility is required to record all work-related injuries and illnesses on the OSHA 200 Log. By collecting and analyzing these logs, you can uncover a wealth of information about the health and safety issues in your facility.

The third chapter focuses on principles for prevention of a number of health and safety issues and includes tips for moving a health and safety agenda forward in your workplace.

Not only do nurses have rights within the workplace, they also have responsibilities. Learning the policies and procedures designed to address their concerns, using the engineering controls in place for their protection and helping to develop new standards for prevention builds not only a healthier and safer working environment but also a strong foundation for nurses' advocacy role.

Nurses across the country are working with their state nurses' associations (constituent members of the American Nurses Association) to provide high-quality patient care, without jeopardizing their own health. Every day, nurses are gaining new victories, whether state passage of legislation for safe needle devices, OSHA inspection ofa facility with poor indoor air quality, new personal protective equipment to prevent exposure to tuberculosis, or increased staffing on a unit with frequent back injuries.

Now is the time to join your state nurses' association, a constituent member of the ANA, partners in creating work environments where risking your life is never an expected "part of the job."

The ANA and all fifty-four Constituent Member Associations are committed to improving the occupational safety and health of registered nurses. ANA works to improve the health and safety of nurses in many ways, including education, federal legislation, state legislation, regulation, and workplace advocacy. For more information on ANA's occupational safety and health program visit ANA's web site: www.nursingworld.org/dlwa/osh.

1

KNOW YOUR RIGHTS

Reports of violence in the workplace, life-threatening latex allergies, and exposure to resistant tuberculosis and nontreatable Hepatitis C are alarming to any nurse. The resulting deaths, injuries, and permanent disabilities are unacceptable.

Although the health care industry is a dangerous place to work, many of the risks are avoidable, and dangerous exposures are preventable. Prevention is key. With up-to-date information and attention to health and safety programs, dangerous environmental and substance exposures can be eliminated!

You can be an effective advocate and partner in providing a safer and healthier work environment. Start by reading this chapter which outlines the privileges and protections OSHA provides to all workers. This guide walks you through the process of identifying and controlling potential hazards in your workplace. You will learn what action to take when you suspect that there is an occupational health and safety problem at your facility. You will also learn how to ensure that your facility adheres to the laws and how to enlist the help of state and federal agencies. It is one thing to know what your rights are under the law; it is quite another to ensure that the facility fulfills its responsibility to provide a safe and healthy workplace. You and your colleagues can work together to ensure that your employer addresses your health and safety concerns.

Hazards in the Health Care Environment: Identification and Control

Reactions to workplace hazards vary from mild symptoms to serious and life-threatening injuries or illnesses, which can lead to permanent disability or even death. For example, 38 percent of all RNs sustain back injuries, which are sometimes career-ending. Every year there are approximately 1,000 new cases of health care workers with HIV, Hepatitis B, or Hepatitis C.

How can you determine which safety and health hazards are causing injuries or illnesses where you work? What can you do about it? The first step is to identify the hazards. The second is to control them.

Identifying Workplace Hazards

Safety and health hazards in the health care workplace fall into the following categories:

■ **Biological hazards** — Bacteria such as TB, viruses such as varicella, fungi or parasites, bloodborne pathogens such as HIV, and Hepatitis B and C. These can be transmitted by contact with infected patients or contaminated body secretions/fluids.

■ **Ergonomic hazards** — Lifting and transferring patients or equipment, or standing for long periods of time, or enduring repetitive strain. These can result in musculoskeletal injuries.

■ **Chemical hazards** — Medications, solutions, and gases such as ethylene oxide, formaldehyde, glutaraldehyde, waste anesthetic gases, laser smoke, cytotoxic agents, pentamidine, and latex.

■ **Psychological hazards** — Shift rotation, stress, and mandatory overtime.

■ **Physical hazards** — Radiation, lasers, noise, and electricity.

Conducting a Walk-Through

A walk-through, which is a workplace inspection, is the first step in identifying hazards, and it serves several important functions. While on a walk-through, hazards can be recognized and often corrected before anyone's health or safety is affected. Talking with workers about the hazards which they face can make them more aware of dangerous conditions and encourage them to become involved in prevention activities. A walk-through is also useful for investigating newly reported hazards.

A workplace walk-through can be conducted by a facility's health and safety committee, as part of an OSHA inspection, or even by you. Walk-throughs should be done once a month during work hours. Walk through all the units and note as many hazards as possible. Speak with supervisors and frontline workers in each department and ask any additional questions that may arise. For example, have common health problems been noticed among the workers in a specific department? Are there any new hazards? How is the given department different from a typical department of its type? A diagram of each department, including the number and location of workers and the sources of potential exposure, should be developed.

Tips for Conducting a Walk-through

■ **Be alert**. Use your senses of sight, smell and hearing as you walk around. Be sensitive to how you and others in the facility feel while working.

■ **Make a diagram**, or get a floor plan of your workplace. Use it to mark hazards and potential risks.

■ **Take notes**. Record the hazard, its location and who is affected. Record whether it occurs continually or at special times.

- **Get a list of hazardous drugs and chemicals** used in the workplace and copies of MSDSs (see page 11) covering the chemicals used in the areas which you will be inspecting.
- **Write a summary report**. Submit a copy to management and to the health and safety committee. Request that action be taken when necessary.

Controlling Workplace Hazards

Once existing and potential hazards in the hospital have been recognized, employees at risk have been identified, and existing control measures have been evaluated, the next step is to assess the need for prevention, control, and/or personal protective equipment. Remember that your facility's occupational health department can be a great source of information and may be a strong ally. Their job, and their professional responsibility, is to promote the health and safety of workers.

Many facilities have Occupational and Environmental Health Nurses/Employee Health Nurses. According to the American Association of Occupational Health Nurses, their role "focuses on the promotion, protection, and restoration of workers' health within the context of a safe and healthy work environment." They are good resources and partners in this process.

Methods to control hazards are usually discussed in terms of the "hierarchy of controls," presented below in descending order of effectiveness, i.e., from most to least effective.

Hierarchy of Controls

Most Effective

- **Elimination** of hazardous materials and dangerous activities, such as the use of needle-less IV systems.

- **Substitution** for less hazardous materials and systems, such as the use of a Steris system to replace glutaraldehyde.

- **Engineering controls**; that is, technical means to isolate or remove hazards from the workplace, such as lifting devices or safer needle devices (for example, needles that sheath, blunt or retract after use).

- **Administrative controls**; that is, policies which limit workers' exposure to hazards, such as appropriate allocation of resources to provide for health and safety program, staffing, and equipment.

- **Work practice controls**, such as no-recapping, and staff assistance for lifting.

- **Personal Protective Equipment (PPE)**, such as barriers and filters between the worker and the hazard (gloves, masks, gowns, etc.).

Least Effective

3

List of OSHA Standards That Apply to Health Care

- ■ Occupational Exposure to Bloodborne Pathogens Standard (29 CFR 1910.1030)
- ■ Hazard Communications Standard (29 CFR 1910.1200)
- ■ Access to Employee Exposure and Medical Records (29 CFR 1910.20)
- ■ Occupational Exposure to Ethylene Oxide (29 CFR 1910.1047)
- ■ Formaldehyde Permissible Exposure Limit (PEL)

Proposed OSHA Standards

- ■ Tuberculosis (enforceable under the General Duty Clause)
- ■ Glutaraldehyde Permissible Exposure Limit (PEL)
- ■ Health and Safety Programs
- ■ Indoor Air

Visit www.osha.gov for more information.

OSHA Protections Mandated by Law

What Is OSHA?

The Occupational Safety and Health Act, or the OSH Act, was passed in 1970, after workers and organizations such as ANA lobbied for improved safety and health conditions at work. The Act created the Occupational Safety and Health Administration (OSHA).

The OSH Act applies to every private employer with one or more employees and assures "every [private-sector] working man and woman a safe and healthful workplace."

OSHA protection also exists for federal employees, and for *some* state and local government employees.

- ■ The OSH Act requires the head of each federal agency (such as the Veterans Administration) to establish and maintain an effective and comprehensive occupational safety and health program consistent with OSHA standards.

- ■ OSHA protection also applies to those state and local government employees who have OSHA-approved occupational safety and health plans (see What Are OSHA-approved State Plans? on page 7).

- ■ *Note:* Public employees without an OSHA-approved state plan are *not* covered by OSHA.

OSHA, part of the U.S. Department of Labor, is responsible for enforcing the OSH Act by setting safety and health standards and by conducting workplace inspections. Employers must comply with OSHA standards or risk being cited and fined for violating the law. **The Joint Commission for the Accreditation of Healthcare Organizations (JCAHO) also requires compliance with OSHA standards.**

OSHA can issue citations for hazardous working conditions. For example, in federal workplaces, OSHA issues a "Notice of Unsafe or Unhealthful Working Conditions." OSHA also can fine employers for hazardous working conditions. On request, OSHA provides consultation services and training classes through local offices on how to comply with OSHA standards, how to create an effective health and safety program, and eliminate specific hazards in the workplace. In some states, these functions are performed by the OSHA-approved state plan.

For more information about your private-sector workplace rights under the OSH Act, read *OSHA: Employee Workplace Rights* (OSHA publication 3021, 1994), which highlights many of the issues discussed below. The rights of federal employees are similar; however, see title 29, Code of Federal Regulations, part 1960 of the OSH Act.

What Are Your Employer's Responsibilities under the OSH Act?

Section 8 of the OSH Act requires your employer to give you a place of employment that is "free from recognized hazards that are causing or are likely to cause death or serious physical harm." Additionally, your employer must "comply with occupational safety and health standards."

What Are Your Rights under the OSH Act?

Under the OSH Act, your employer must:

- let you know about the OSHA safety and health standards that apply to your workplace;

- give you a copy of those standards and the OSHA law itself;

- tell you about the safety and health hazards in your workplace, the precautions that you can take to protect yourself, and the procedures to follow if you are involved in an accident or exposed to a toxic substance;

- give you access to your exposure and medical records;

- allow you to observe any monitoring or measuring of hazardous materials in your workplace and see the resulting records; and

- give you access to the company's OSHA Form No.200, Log and Summary of Occupational Injuries and Illnesses, known as the OSHA 200 Log, or the federal agency equivalent.

OSHA Guidelines that Apply to Health Care

- OSHA Technical Manual: Controlling Occupational Exposure to Hazardous Drugs (TED 1-0.15A)

- Ergonomic Guidelines For Meatpacking Plants (OSHA 3123)

- Guidelines For Preventing Workplace Violence For Health Care And Social Service Workers (OSHA 3148)

OSHA may cite and fine, under the General Duty Clause, for violating OSHA guidelines. **Visit www.osha.gov for more information.**

5

Note: Beginning January 1, 2002, OSHA's new recordkeeping rule, which was issued on January 19, 2001 as a revision of their old recordkeeping rule (29 CFR 1904), will be enforced. Under the new rule, employers will be required to record and keep work-related injury and illness information on an **OSHA 300 Log.**

What Can OSHA Do about Unsafe or Unhealthy Working Conditions?

OSHA can provide the following services.

Inspect, Cite, and Fine

OSHA, or the OSHA-approved state plan administrators, can inspect the workplace and issue citations to your employer for violating standards set under the OSH Act. If no standard exists for a particular hazard (such as for lifting or repetitive motion that can cause neck and back injuries) or if there are only OSH guidelines, OSHA may issue a citation under the OSH Act's General Duty Clause (www.osha.gov/OshAct).

General Duty Clause Violation

You and your colleagues may have to help OSHA build a case for a General Duty Clause citation. You must show that the hazard exists. The OSHA 200 log (see Chapter 2), health and safety committee minutes, grievance complaints, and workers' compensation paid will be valuable evidence of the hazard. You also will need to show that:

■ the hazard is causing or is likely to cause serious physical harm or death,

■ there are effective methods to control the hazard, and

■ these control methods are feasible.

If cited, your employer must post the written citation where employees can see it. Look for the citation in your workplace and make certain that it is posted for the entire time required on the citation. The citation will describe the violation and give your employer a deadline for correcting the problem. Besides issuing the citation, OSHA also may fine your employer.

Your employer may appeal the citation and fine. You and your colleagues may object to your employer's appeal; however, your objection must be in writing within 15 days of your employer's filing of this appeal.

Can an Exception Be Made for Your Employer?

The OSH Act (part 1905) gives your employer the right to apply for a variance, which is an alternative to following an OSHA standard. (Federal agencies may request "alternate standards" under OSHA 29 CFR 1960.) Applying for a variance does not remove your employer's responsibility to "provide for employment and place of employment which are as safe and healthful as those required by the standard for which a variance is sought," as stated in the OSH Act.

Your employer must notify you that it has sought a variance and must post a copy of the application in the workplace where employees can see it. You and your colleagues have the right to request a hearing about your employer's request for a variance.

What Are OSHA-approved State Plans?

Under the OSH Act, section 18, individual states can apply to develop and administer their own safety and health plans. This federally approved OSHA coverage is administered by the state and also covers public employees. If an OSHA standard exists for a hazard, the state's safety and health standard for that hazard must be *at least as effective as* the OSHA standard. If federal standards do not address a hazard, the state may issue its own standards. Currently, 25 states and territories administer their own programs through OSHA-approved state plans.

If your state has an OSHA-approved state plan, direct all your inquiries or complaints directly to the agency administering the plan. Work with your SNA to lobby for protective legislation or regulation such as safer needle devices or a latex allergy standard. Visit ANA's web site, www.nursingworld.org for sample legislation language. Your state plan, like the federal OSHA, enforces the standards that it sets and provides free consultation services.

See Appendix D for a complete listing of OSHA-approved state plans or visit OSHA's Internet site at www.osha.gov for an up-to-date directory.

Can I Refuse Unsafe Work?

The OSH Act specifically states that you cannot be discriminated against for refusing unsafe work; this is known as the "Imminent Danger" provision of the Act. The conditions necessary to justify a work refusal are very stringent. As a result, refusing unsafe work should be a last resort. If you are confronted by a hazard in your workplace that poses an imminent danger of death or serious injury:

- Inform your employer and request that the hazard be corrected immediately;
- Ask that no workers be exposed to the hazardous condition until the danger has been eliminated or controlled;
- Document the circumstances of the hazardous condition;
- Offer to perform other work while the hazard is being corrected; and
- Contact OSHA and request an immediate inspection if your employer refuses to act.

Clearly, it is better to be fired than to be seriously injured or killed, but do not refuse work under the illusion that there is strong legal protection. For those who have refused work and were then fired, reinstatement in their jobs, if ever, has taken months or even years.

Before there is a dangerous situation, understand your employee rights that allow you to refuse work under certain conditions. Also work with your state nurses' association to understand your state laws and regulations.

The OSH Act, the National Labor Relations Act, and the union grievance-arbitration process can reinstate a worker who has been discriminated against for refusal to work under unsafe conditions. The legal system requires that the following conditions be met for granting reinstatement:

- The employer gives the worker no alternative to either working under unsafe conditions or refusing work;

- The employer denies the request to correct the hazard before requiring work to continue;

- The hazard is such that any reasonable person would, under similar circumstances, reach the same conclusion; and,

- The danger is such that there is not enough time to wait for an OSHA inspection.

Under the National Labor Relations Act, certain other criteria, such as refusing dangerous work in cooperation with or on behalf of other workers, may apply. *This protection applies to any concerted activity at work, whether you are in a union or not.* Contact your SNA or the National Labor Relations Board for more information.

Is There Whistleblower Protection?

Whistleblower protection is protection from punishment for speaking out against unsafe or illegal practices in the workplace. Section 11(c) of the OSH Act empowers you to exercise your OSHA rights without fear of discrimination or discharge from employment. If you believe that you have been punished for your actions (for example, for filing a grievance or complaining about your employer to OSHA or any other government agency about job safety and health hazards, or for participating in OSHA inspections, hearings, or other OSHA-related activities), you should contact the nearest OSHA office within 30 days after you learn of the discriminatory act. If OSHA finds that your complaint has merit, your employer must reinstate your employment and pay:

- back pay;

- related compensation;

- compensatory damages; and

- your expenses for bringing the complaint.

See section 11(c) of the OSH Act for more details about the complaint/appeal process. Other whistle-blower protections, most specifically related to the concerted refusal of hazardous work, are found in the National Labor Relations Act. Individual states also afford protections related to retaliation for speaking out against your employer. Federal agency employees are given protection against retaliation under OSHA 29 CFR 1960.

What Can OSHA Do in Addition to Enforcing Regulation?

OSHA consultation services and cooperative programs are two additional agency resources.

OSHA Consultation Services

Under the OSH Act (OSHA 29 CFR 1908), private-sector employers may obtain free safety and health consultation services through either the local OSHA office or the OSHA-approved state plan. However, for federal agencies, there may be some cost.

OSHA's consultation services, which include education and training for employers and workers, are intended to help employers prevent occupational injuries and illnesses. For the most part, OSHA provides consultation services at the work site, but off-site consultation may be provided by telephone, through correspondence, or at the local OSHA office. OSHA sets its priorities for consultation services on the basis of industry hazards and business (or agency) size, with smaller organizations having higher priority.

If OSHA finds a hazard during a consultation visit, your employer must agree to remove the hazard. All records and documentation provided by the OSHA officer are accessible to you under the Freedom of Information Act and the OSH Act's Access to Employee Exposure and Medical Records Standard (OSHA 29 CFR 1910.20).

Cooperative Programs

Your employer may choose to participate in one of OSHA's programs that offers special considerations in return for cooperative agreements with OSHA. Ask your employer whether it is involved in Voluntary Protection Programs (VPPs), Cooperative Compliance Programs, or other OSHA initiatives. Most programs provide for increased employee participation in safety and health.

Caution: Be aware that VPP employers will not experience routine inspections, and that OSHA inspections in VPP workplaces will only occur in response to a complaint. Work together with your facility's Health and Safety committee to evaluate the success of the VPP and how best to ensure compliance.

NIOSH

The 1970 OSH Act also created NIOSH, the National Institute for Occupational Safety and Health as part of the Centers for Disease Control and Prevention (CDC) within the U.S. Department of Health and Human Services. NIOSH is the only federal institute responsible for conducting research and recommending ways to prevent work-related injuries and illnesses. NIOSH's responsibilities include:

- investigating potentially hazardous working conditions, if requested;

- evaluating workplace hazards;

- creating and disseminating innovative methods, techniques, and approaches for dealing with occupational safety and health problems;

- conducting research and making recommendations related to the development of occupational safety and health standards; and

- providing training programs to increase the number and competence of personnel working in occupational safety and health.

NIOSH Health Hazard Evaluation

NIOSH has no enforcement authority. However, NIOSH does have the authority, under section 20 of the OSH Act, to conduct a health hazard evaluation (HHE) when requested by an employer, or an employee, with the signatures of two additional employees. At times, filing an OSHA complaint is a more appropriate action than requesting an HHE. If you have questions about which action is appropriate, contact your state nurses' association.

You are protected against discrimination for requesting an HHE. Additionally, you can ask to have your name withheld from the documentation of your request for an HHE. Any personnel information gathered during an HHE is safeguarded in accordance with the 1974 Privacy Act.

Since your employer neither pays for nor controls an HHE, it may offer an unbiased evaluation. Among the reasons to request an HHE from NIOSH are:

■ employees have an illness from an unknown cause;

■ employees are exposed to an agent or working condition that is not regulated by OSHA;

■ employees experience negative health effects from exposure to a chemical, physical agent, or working condition, even though the legal limit is not being exceeded;

■ medical or epidemiological investigations are needed to evaluate the hazard;

■ the occurrence of a particular disease or injury is higher than expected in a group of employees;

■ the exposure is to a new or previously unrecognized hazard, technology, or piece of equipment; or

■ the hazard seems to be resulting from the combined effects of several agents.

During an HHE, NIOSH may:

■ observe work practices and conduct industrial hygiene exposure monitoring, medical tests, or physical exams;

■ conduct confidential interviews with employees; or

■ review workplace exposure, medical, and OSHA 200 Log records.

You have the right to accompany NIOSH when it initially inspects your workplace, as well as during the opening and closing conferences with management. NIOSH will give you copies of all reports. Additionally, your employer must post the final report where all workers can have access to it.

NIOSH Publications

NIOSH publishes various documents based on its own research and on summaries of research performed by others. Among them are:

■ **NIOSH Alerts**, which briefly present new information about occupational illnesses, injuries, and deaths, and urge assistance in preventing, solving, and controlling newly identified occupational safety and health hazards. Examples include Preventing Allergic Reaction to Natural Rubber Latex in the Workplace, and Preventing Needlestick Injuries in Health Care Settings.

■ **NIOSH Criteria Documents**, which contain critical reviews of the scientific and technical information available on the existence of safety and health risks and hazards, along with the adequacy of methods to identify and control them.

- **Current Intelligence Bulletins**, which review and evaluate new and emerging information about occupational hazards, including newly identified hazards, new information on known hazards, and hazard controls.

- **Special Hazard Reviews and Occupational Hazard Assessments**, which assess safety and health problems and recommend appropriate methods for control and monitoring, and which often are used to complement recommendations for OSHA standards.

- **Joint Occupational Health Documents**, which are developed with foreign government agencies.

NIOSH publications are free and available on request. To order, call 1–800–35–NIOSH or visit www.cdc.gov/niosh. See Appendix H for a listing of health care worker related publications.

Education Research Centers

NIOSH currently funds 15 university sites, called Education Research Centers (ERCs), to train personnel in occupational safety and health fields and to provide community safety and health education courses. ERC personnel can be valuable resources for you. See Appendix I for a list of ERC contacts.

NIOSH ERCs also fund graduate study in occupational health nursing.

What Is the "Right to Know"?

You have a legal right to know—so exercise your rights. OSHA's Hazard Communication Standard (OSHA 29 CFR 1910.1200) is known as the "right to know." It gives you legal rights to obtain information on chemical hazards in your workplace. It requires your employer to have a written plan to:

- identify the hazardous chemicals that you may be exposed to,

- give you access to information about those chemicals,

- train you in the health effects of exposure to the chemicals and in methods of using them properly,

- list all chemicals found in each department in your workplace and make that list available to all employees on all shifts, and

- provide Material Safety Data Sheets (MSDSs), which include safety and health information about each chemical.

Analyzing the Material Safety Data Sheets (MSDSs)

Material Safety Data Sheets (MSDSs) provide basic information about chemicals used in your facility. Employers are required to provide the MSDSs to employees, and they must be kept in a readily accessible location at each work site. The chemical manufacturer or importer of the hazardous chemical product produces the MSDS.

An MSDS includes the following types of information:

- chemical name and trade name of the product

- manufacturer's name, address, and emergency telephone number

- hazardous ingredients in the product

- physical and chemical characteristics of the chemical

- data on the fire and explosion characteristics of the chemical

- data on the reactivity of the chemical with other materials, byproducts, etc

- health hazard information, such as routes of entry, effects of exposure, signs and symptoms of exposure

- emergency and first aid procedures

- personal protective equipment or ventilation requirements for using the product

- other precautions for safe handling and use, such as disposal of wastes, storage, and spill information

Make sure that the MSDS is available on all units where the following chemicals are used or stored: glutaraldehyde (Cidex), paracetic acid (used in Steris machines), cleaning agents, ethylene oxide, formaldehyde, antineoplastic drugs, mercury, asbestos, methyl methacrylate (glue for joint replacement), and for any other chemical used in the workplace.

How to Read a Material Safety Data Sheet

MSDSs can be very useful, if they are accurate and complete. The following paragraphs describe each section of an MSDS.

Section I — Material Identification

This section should include the chemical's identity or trade name (the name which the manufacturer gives to the product), along with the name, address, and emergency telephone number of the manufacturer. Compare that information to the product's container label—they should match. The date on which the MSDS was prepared should also be documented. MSDSs that are more than three years old may contain outdated information and may need to be replaced with a current MSDS.

Section II — Hazardous Ingredients/Identification Information

Since the product may be a mixture of chemicals, the MSDS lists the name of each chemical found in the mixture. Depending on differing requirements in state laws, some chemicals found in the product may *not* be listed, only those required. Usually the chemicals listed are those determined in studies to be toxic.

In addition, the Chemical Abstract Services (CAS) number is listed. The CAS number differentiates among chemicals with similar names; this is useful information when looking up specific chemicals in resource manuals. The OSHA PEL (Permissible Exposure Limit—the legal limit), ACGIH (American

Conference of Governmental Industrial Hygienists) TLV (Threshold Limit Values—recommended limit), and other show the acceptable or legal amounts of a chemical to which workers can be exposed without expected health problems.

Section III — Physical/Chemical Characteristics

This section describes the various properties of a chemical that will affect its potential for causing harm to a person using the product.

- **Boiling Point** is the temperature at which a liquid chemical boils or becomes a gas. The lower the number, the quicker the substance will evaporate and put potentially harmful vapors into the air. Any chemical with a boiling point below 100 degrees Celsius (212 degrees Fahrenheit) requires special caution.

- **Vapor Pressure** is another indication of a chemical's evaporation speed. The higher the vapor pressure, the more easily and quickly the liquid chemical evaporates and can be inhaled.

- **Vapor Density** describes how easily the chemical, once evaporated, rises into the air. A vapor density less than 1 tends to rise; a vapor density greater than 1 tends to fall. This information is important for identifying emergency escape procedures, such as whether to drop to the floor and crawl out, if the vapor density is less than 1.

- **Appearance and Odor** help to identify the substance. However, be aware that many chemicals may have similar colors. In addition, some chemicals are hazardous at levels lower than those at which they can be smelled. Other chemicals cause olfactory fatigue, which means that you lose the ability to smell the chemical after a short time. This information is helpful in case of spills, leaks or accidents involving unfamiliar chemicals.

- **Specific Gravity** describes the tendency of a chemical to sink or float in water. In general, a specific gravity greater than 1 indicates that the chemical will sink in water; a specific gravity of less than 1 indicates that the chemical will float in water.

- **Evaporation Rate** is similar to vapor pressure. It is the rate at which a chemical evaporates compared with another substance. Butyl acetate is a chemical that evaporates very slowly and is commonly used as a comparison substance. If the chemical has an evaporation rate greater than 1, it evaporates faster than the substance with which it is compared.

Section IV — Fire and Explosion Hazard Data

Fire and explosion hazard data provide helpful information for determining the flammability of the chemical and any special precautions that are necessary in case of a fire.

- **Flash Point** is the lowest temperature at which a liquid chemical ignites. Chemicals with flash points below 100 degrees Fahrenheit are considered flammable; those with flash points between 100 and 200 degrees Fahrenheit are considered combustible. Such chemicals require special handling and storage precautions.

- **Extinguishing Media** describes the kinds of fire extinguishers to use with a fire involving the particular chemicals.

■ **Special Fire-Fighting Procedures** and **Unusual Fire and Explosion Hazards** further describe the types of extinguishing equipment and fire-fighting approaches. These procedures should protect the safety of those fighting a fire involving the chemical.

Section V — Reactivity Data

The reactions of chemicals when mixed with other chemicals or materials are described in this section. The information should be used to avoid explosions and other dangerous reactions.

Section VI — Health Hazard Data

This section describes the health effects which these chemicals may cause, including the signs and symptoms of exposure, medical conditions made worse by exposure to the chemical, the body organs that the chemical affects, which effects are acute or chronic, and whether the chemical causes cancer or birth defects.

This section should tell whether the chemical is:

■ a corrosive (physical contact with the chemical causes the gradual eating or wearing away of a substance, particularly the skin),

■ an irritant (exposure causes an excessive response to stimulation, such as sneezing after breathing a chemical), or

■ a sensitizer (exposure causes an allergic type of reaction, making individuals more sensitive to the chemical the next time they are exposed).

The route of exposure, i.e., how the chemical enters the body, is listed as inhalation, skin contact, or ingestion/swallowing.

Section VII — Precautions for Safe Handling and Use

Information on the type of equipment to use when handling, storing, or cleaning up a chemical leak or spill is given in this section. The proper way to dispose of the chemical should also be listed.

Section VIII — Control Measures

This section gives recommendations to ensure a safe work environment while using the chemical. Included here are control measures such as engineering designs (proper ventilation systems) or safe work practices, as well as the type of personal protective equipment to use.

MSDS Quick Check

The MSDS lists a great deal of information, which may make it difficult to determine how hazardous a product actually is. Here is a quick MSDS checklist:

❑ Look in the Hazardous Ingredients section to see whether the chemical is listed.

❑ Look for signal words such as "danger" or "warning" which indicate hazardous chemicals.

❑ Chemicals with PELs less than 25 ppm or TLVs less than 2 mg/cubic meter are more hazardous at lower levels of exposure.

❏ The abbreviations NTP, IARC, A, or A2 indicate that the chemical is a known or suspected cancer-causing agent.

❏ A boiling point less than 100 degrees Celsius (212 degrees Fahrenheit) or flash point less than 60 degrees Celsius (140 degrees Fahrenheit) is more hazardous.

❏ Any mention of cancer; reproductive problems; nerve, liver, or kidney problems; allergy or sensitization; or words such as toxic or "harmful by inhalation or skin contact" should alert you that this chemical is hazardous.

❏ In the section on precautions for safe handling and use, hazardous chemicals are indicated by warnings such as "do not breathe;" "if inhaled, remove to fresh air;" "avoid skin contact;" or "for skin contact, wash immediately."

Exposure Monitoring

During a work site analysis, when identifying existing and potential hazards, exposure monitoring is used to evaluate the worker's level of exposure to a specific chemical agent, such as ethylene oxide (EtO) a cold sterilizing agent. Exposure monitoring must be measured when the chemical is being used. OSHA sets exposure limits, called Permissible Exposure Limits (PELs), for the safe amount of a specific air contaminant and the duration of the exposure. Exposure monitoring is required to determine whether PELs have been exceeded. Adverse effects are still possible at exposure levels lower than those specified by OSHA—and not all toxic chemicals have had limits set. For example, the cold sterilizing agent glutaraldehyde does not have a PEL, despite evidence collected since 1991 demonstrating the need for exposure controls. ANA is lobbying OSHA to publish a PEL for glutaraldehyde.

Recommendations about occupational exposure limits are also available from NIOSH (National Institute for Occupational Safety and Health) and the American Conference of Governmental Industrial Hygienists (ACGIH). Their recommended exposure limits, while not required under law, are useful in evaluating risk (see Appendix H).

What Additional Information about Chemical Hazards Can Be Requested?

You can submit a written request to NIOSH for information on potentially toxic substances in your workplace. You have the right to ask that your name be withheld from your employer. More importantly, you may request that your employer provide more information about chemical hazards and toxic exposures found in your workplace. See Figure 1-1 for a sample letter on requesting information about chemical hazards and toxic exposures. Your request must be in writing and should indicate:

■ to whom to release the information,

■ for whom the information is being requested,

■ why you are requesting the information, and

■ how long you or your representative require access to the information.

FIGURE 1-1. SAMPLE LETTER FOR RELEASE OF EXPOSURE AND CHEMICAL HAZARD RECORDS

[Date]

[Company]
[Address]

Subject: Exposure and chemical hazard records

Dear [name of company manager]:

Pursuant to OSHA's Hazard Communication Standard (OSHA CFR 1910.1200) and the Access to Employee Exposure and Medical Records Standard (OSHA CFR 1910.20) or corresponding state regulations, I am requesting copies of:

____   A list of all toxic chemicals used in my work location.

___   The results of any exposure monitoring conducted in my work location, including my past or present exposure to toxic substances, harmful physical agents, noise, or heat. I am also requesting exposure records for other employees with past or present duties or working conditions related to or similar to mine. Additionally, I am requesting records containing exposure information concerning my workplace or working conditions.

___   Any records of analysis using the above exposure data.

___   Copies of Material Safety Data Sheets that you have on file for chemicals used in my work location.

____   A copy of your written hazard communication program.

I understand that, in compliance with OSHA standards CFR 1910.1200 and CFR 1910.20 or corresponding state regulations, I will be given copies of this information or the opportunity to copy it myself, within 15 days, at a convenient time and place.

Sincerely,

[Signature]
[Your name]
[Address]
[Telephone number]

cc: [Your state nurses association]

Under the OSH Act's Hazard Communication Standard (OSHA 29 CFR 1910.1200), your employer may refuse to provide the information that you request, claiming that the chemical make-up of the substance is a "trade secret." In other words, your employer believes that revealing the ingredients of the substance would give competitors an unfair advantage. However, your employer must still give you information about the characteristics of the chemical and its potential health effects. Additionally, your healthcare provider may have access to the actual chemical name if it is needed for your medical treatment.

Note: Federal agencies may withhold chemical information if disclosure might threaten national security.

Access to Medical Records and Exposure Data

Exposure, medical, and other types of records can tell you whether you are exposed to hazardous materials that may affect your health—now or in the future. Industrial hygiene samples and biological monitoring results can tell you whether the engineering controls and personal protective equipment in your workplace are functioning properly and preventing injuries and illnesses. Reports of workplace inspections and accident reports can help you to locate areas where problems already have been identified. This information can help you to identify areas in your workplace or certain job tasks that may have exposures.

Your own medical records can tell you what effects noise, chemicals, or radiation may be having on your health. Records of groups of employees can help you to identify patterns of workplace injuries or illnesses. Your state nurses' association may be able to use those records to show that a health problem is a larger workplace problem and not limited to just one person.

Exposure and medical records may contain technical information. You may want to consult with a trusted healthcare provider or other qualified professionals from your state nurses' association who are knowledgeable in occupational exposures and related health problems.

Use the information that you access to identify and document workplace hazards and hazardous conditions and to develop connections between job exposure and injury/illness occurrence. You can then bring that information to management's attention and to OSHA's attention also, if necessary. Again, work with your state nurses' association for guidance and direction for proper reporting.

The OSH Act's Access to Employee Exposure and Medical Records Standard (OSHA 29 CFR 1910.20) gives you the right to see exposure and medical records, including any analyses of the information in those records. The law applies to all employee exposure and medical records, whether or not those records are required by specific occupational safety and health standards. It also applies to records made or maintained either in-house or through a contractual company.

When requesting access to records, it is best to do so in writing, making sure that the request is dated. Although OSHA allows verbal requests, written requests provide documentation for future reference especially if any legal action is necessary.

Medical Records

You also have the right to request a copy of the medical records kept by your employer (see Figure 1-2). Your employer must tell you when you are first hired, and then at least annually, how you can access your medical records. Your employer must keep your medical records for at least 30 years after you leave employment.

Your medical records should include the following:

- medical histories and questionnaires;
- laboratory test results;
- medical exam results;
- medical opinions, diagnoses, and recommendations;
- worker medical complaints;
- original X-rays, including interpretations;
- descriptions of treatments and prescriptions; and
- records about health insurance claims, if accessible to the employer by employee name or personal ID number.

Exposure Records

You have the right to see the results of any exposure monitoring that has been conducted in your work area. Your employer must tell you, when you are first hired, and then at least annually:

- that exposure monitoring records exist,
- where exposure records are located, and
- how you can access exposure records.

Exposure records should include the following:

- industrial hygiene sampling data,
- biological monitoring tests for toxic chemicals, and,
- MSDSs or other records that identify toxic substances or harmful physical agents in your work area.

Your employer must keep all exposure records for at least 30 years after the date of the test or procedure used to produce the records.

Group Records or Aggregate Data

You are guaranteed access to "any compilation of data or any research, statistical or other study" that your employer has prepared from exposure data or medical records. Your employer must give you that information after deleting all personal identifying information.

Workers' Compensation Records

Workers' compensation laws are determined by state governments, not OSHA. Federal agencies are governed by the Office of Workers' Compensation Program (OWCP).

Figure 1-2. Sample Letter for Release of Employee Medical Records

[Date]

[Company]
[Address]

Subject: Release of employee medical records

Dear [name of company manager]:

Pursuant to OSHA's Access to Employee Exposure and Medical Records Standard (OSHA CFR 1910.20) or corresponding state regulations, I hereby authorize [name of company] to release the following medical information from my personal medical records, whether kept by the company or its consultants:

____   Medical and employment questionnaires and histories.
____   Results of medical exams and laboratory tests.
____   Medical opinions, diagnoses, progress notes, and recommendations.
____   Descriptions of treatment and prescriptions.
____   Medical complaints.
____   Health insurance claims records that can be retrieved by personal identifier.
____   Any records of analyses done using employee medical data.
____   Other _____

I give my permission for this medical information to be used for the following purposes: [Describe the approved use of these records; for example, diagnosing, treating, and compensating occupational disease or analysis of workplace hazards]. I do not give my [ermission for any other use or re-disclosure of this information. This release is effective until this date: [date]

Sincerely,

[Signature]
[Your name]
[Address]
[Telephone number]

cc: [Your state nurses association]

The workers' compensation system was created to provide "no-fault" compensation to workers who are injured or die on the job. Benefits include a percentage of wage replacement, medical costs, and costs of rehabilitation. Your employer must pay the benefits, regardless of who is at fault. You do not have to prove that your employer was negligent. For more information about the laws governing your workplace, contact your state workers' compensation board, or, if you are a federal employee, the OWCP.

Your state's workers' compensation board (or the OWCP) keeps records on individual worker claims, along with full records for your workplace and group data on types of injuries and illnesses that have occurred each year. Some of that information is available to you as a matter of public record.

However, workers' compensation claims are considered health insurance claims under the OSH Act's Access to Employee Exposure and Medical Records Standard (OSHA 29 CFR 1910.20) and may not be accessible to you. Contact your state workers' compensation board (or OWCP) for more information about releasing your personal or group records.

Other Records and Data

Additional records from OSHA, the U.S. Environmental Protection Agency (EPA), NIOSH, and other government agencies related to safety and health in your workplace are available to you through the Freedom of Information Act. Congress passed the Freedom of Information Act in 1966, giving the public access to information held by the federal government. Additionally, most states have their own laws governing disclosure of records to the public. The 1974 Privacy Act limits what information may be released. To request records from government agencies, you must give your reasons for wanting the records. Some fees may be charged for the records.

Taking Action

Once you identify the hazards in your workplace and learn about your rights under OSHA, you can take action in many ways to improve the health and safety of your workplace! The following section outlines specific steps that you can take to make positive changes and improve the health and safety of your workplace.

Document, Document, Document!

All nurses have a responsibility to document. Documentation is always the first step, and it is essential that you and your colleagues report and document every occupational injury and illness in order to:

- collect data to evaluate the health and safety of your workplace;
- collect data that can be used by your SNA and ANA to lobby state and federal agencies for more protections;
- ensure timely post-exposure follow-up, including testing and treatment. For example, if a nurse is stuck with a needle and there is a risk of HIV, post-exposure prophylaxis should begin within two hours of exposure;
- ensure workers' compensation payments;

■ ensure that all health expenses are charged to workers' compensation and not to the individual's health insurance;

■ ensure that any missed days at work due to work-related injuries are counted against workers' compensation and not sick leave or vacation days; and

■ forward the data to OSHA for inclusion in Bureau of Labor Statistics data (these national statistics drive national policy).

The importance of documenting cannot be overstated. Help your colleagues to understand that documenting will improve their safety and health. Promptly reporting a needlestick or other injury also can protect you in the future, if the injury leads to a serious illness. It is in your best interest—no matter how busy you are—to document illnesses and injuries. Needlesticks, for example, are greatly under-reported. If the true number of needlesticks were reported, the astounding figure would most likely spur facilities and state and federal governments into action. Until nurses are constantly and consistently documenting, only estimates can be made.

Health and Safety Committees

Many employment settings have their own occupational safety and health committee, and often this includes an Occupational Health Nurse or Employee Health Nurse. If yours does not, establishing one is a good first step. The safety and health committee can be a valuable source of assistance for safety and health problems in your workplace.

The Joint Commission on Accreditation of Healthcare Organizations (JCAHO) requires that all hospitals have a safety and health committee that meets at least every other month and reports its activities quarterly to specific members of the hospital community, including the governing body and chief executive officer.

Safety and health committee members do not have to be experts in safety and health, but they are experts in the daily work of RNs in your facility. With time and effort, the committee can gather information, document problems, and figure out strategies to address safety and health issues. Nurses and other employees can learn about the hazards in the workplace and help management to correct those hazards.

Your state nurses' association (SNA) is another valuable resource, so inform your SNA about safety and health problems and successes within your facility. As a constituent member of the American Nurses Association, it can assist you and inform you of successful strategies used by RNs across the country.

These committees can help to resolve health and safety problems. A solid committee structure, mutual respect between nurses and management, and an understanding of the importance of safety and health issues, are essential. A good committee will:

■ include equal representation of staff and management,

■ have staff nurse representatives selected by their peers (including affected employees),

■ rotate the committee chair between staff and management,

■ schedule committee meetings at least monthly,

- provide training for the effective participation of committee members,

- prepare and distribute an agenda at least a week before each meeting,

- obtain management commitment to and schedules for correcting unsafe conditions, and document both in the meeting minutes,

- distribute meeting minutes to both staff and management,

- conduct meetings and inspections during regular work hours, paying committee members regular wages for all time spent on committee functions.

The committee can work to improve the health and safety program by:

- identifying workplace safety and health problems—for example, by conducting surveys and walk-throughs, investigating employee complaints or concerns, reviewing work processes, requesting records, and investigating accidents and close calls,

- conducting follow-up inspections to ensure that management follows through on committee recommendations,

- educating other workers about safety and health hazards, and,

- publicizing safety and health problems and solutions by using fact sheets, leaflets, newsletters and bulletin board postings.

If management does not correct committee-identified safety and health hazards, the committee should consider filing an OSHA complaint.

Filing a Complaint with OSHA

If your employer is not meeting its responsibilities and your health is at risk, there are steps that you can take. However, while exercising your rights to protection under the law, it is best to act in concert with a committee, rather than alone. Contact your SNA before you file a complaint with OSHA. Your state nurses' association has access to more information and resources. You have rights to protect your safety and health, and if you speak out about those rights, you are protected—if the proper steps are carefully followed.

While you are not required to discuss concerns with your employer before filing a complaint, when possible, you and your employer should work together to identify hazards and resolve occupational safety and health problems. Documenting the specific OSHA standards being violated and offering possible solutions often helps to convince management to correct hazards. Work with your supervisor and your shared governance or health and safety committee to make your employer aware that you are concerned enough to contact OSHA for an inspection if no action is taken. Of course, if there is imminent danger to life or health, call your local OSHA office STAT!

According to the OSH Act, you may file a complaint by telephone or in writing. If there is no imminent danger, make the complaint in writing.

When Should I File a Complaint with OSHA?

You should file a complaint with OSHA when:

- immediate enforcement action is needed,

- the hazard is one that is well recognized,

■ management has refused to comply with existing occupational safety and health standards, and

■ the OSHA standard is known to adequately protect employees from the hazard.

If you are a federal employee, file your complaint as a "Report of Unsafe or Unhealthful Working Conditions."

See Figure 1-3 for a sample complaint letter. Do not delay filing your complaint even if you do not have all the information. The information which you provide in your complaint will help the OSHA compliance officer determine the seriousness of the hazard and its priority on OSHA's inspection list. If possible, your complaint should include:

■ a clear description of the workplace and its hazards,

■ the number of workers exposed to the hazards,

■ when the hazards occur (ongoing or at specific times),

■ any related injuries or illnesses,

■ the name of the OSHA standard being violated,

■ how long management has known about the hazards, and

■ what actions, if any, management has taken to correct them.

What Are My Rights?

You have the right to:

■ request that OSHA inspect your workplace,

■ accompany the OSHA compliance officer during the inspection,

■ answer any questions that the OSHA compliance officer asks during the inspection,

■ object to the length or conditions of the abatement period set by OSHA for correcting a violation in a citation issued to your employer,

■ submit a written request to NIOSH for information on potentially toxic substances in your workplace,

■ know whether your employer applies for a variance from an OSHA standard (called an "alternate standard" for federal agencies), testifies at a variance hearing, or appeals a final OSHA decision,

■ ask OSHA to withhold your name from your employer if you file a written complaint with OSHA or request information or assistance from NIOSH,

■ know about any decisions that OSHA makes regarding a complaint, and

■ file a section 11(c) discrimination complaint if you are punished for exercising your OSHA rights or for refusing hazardous work if you are in imminent danger of serious injury or death and OSHA has enough time to inspect your workplace. (This is one form of "whistleblower protection.")

To voice an objection about the length or conditions of the abatement period set by OSHA, write to the OSHA area director within 15 working days from

FIGURE 1-3. SAMPLE COMPLAINT LETTER TO OSHA

[Date]

[OSHA area/regional office or state plan office]
[Address]

Subject: Notice of alleged safety or health hazards

Pursuant to my right to file a complaint with OSHA [or my OSHA-approved state plan office], this letter serves as a complaint against the employer named below and as a request for an inspection or other resolution of this issue.

[Employer name]
[Site location: street, city, ZIP code]
[Mailing address, if different]
[Manager or supervisor at the site]
Telephone number at the site]

[Description of the type of business and work at the site]

[Description of the hazard – Describe the alleged hazard in detail, giving as many details as possible, including: who is affected, what the hazard is, where and when the hazard exists, what is causing the hazard, and what the employer has done to eliminate the hazard.]

[Hazard location – Name the specific building or work site.]

This hazard has been brought to the attention of;
      My employer [name the person(s)]
      Other government agency [specify]

[Indicate one of the following with an X.]
____   Do not reveal the names of any of the individuals noted below to this employer.
____   Any of the names of the individuals noted below may be revealed to this employer.

The undersigned believes that a violation of an occupational safety or health standard exists and that it is a job safety or health hazard at the establishment named in this letter.

[Mark an X in the appropriate space(s).]
__ Employee __ Other [identify; for instance, legal counsel]
[Complainant name]
[Telephone number]
[Address – street, city, ZIP code]

[Signature]

cc: [Your state nurses association]

the date when your employer receives the citation. (For federal agency details, see OSHA 29 CFR 1960.)

Participating in an OSHA Inspection

Under OSHA 29 CFR 1903 (and under OSHA 29 CFR 1960 for federal agencies), OSHA has the right to enter the workplace, or any area where work is performed, to inspect and investigate safety and health conditions, equipment, and records. In general, OSHA does not give the employer advance notice. OSHA inspections are carried out:

- as a programmed inspection for high-risk industries or industries with a high incidence of accidents and illnesses, or for review of specific standards,

- in response to a complaint by a worker or worker representative, or

- as a follow-up to a catastrophic accident or death.

Under section 8(e) of the OSH Act, the employee's health and safety representative has a right to accompany the OSHA compliance officer (also referred to as a compliance safety and health officer, CSHO, or inspector) during an inspection, including the initial meeting with the employer, the inspection process itself, and the closing conference. Neither the employer nor the OSHA officer can select the representative.

If you are the representative during an inspection:

- Make sure that the inspector talks with nurses who have knowledge of the health and safety hazards in the workplace. *All workers have the right to speak privately and confidentially with the compliance officer.*

- Point out hazards. Ask the inspector to pay special attention to unsafe needles, sharps containers, or other high risk areas, where injuries or accidents have occurred.

- Report any latex allergy problems and identify the alternatives to powdered latex gloves.

- Report whether N-95 (TB) respirators are available, and, if available, whether they are used when caring for patients with known or suspected TB.

- Point out lifting devices in use, or lack of lifting devices.

- Describe near-misses, injuries, accidents or illnesses which have resulted from uncontrolled hazards. Provide as many facts as possible—the "who, when, where, and how" of work-related incidents.

- Describe past worker complaints.

- If working conditions are not normal during the inspection, tell the inspector. If work is being performed in a safer way than usual, the inspector should know.

- Help the inspector to evaluate employer records on injuries and illnesses.

If you have requested an inspection, you have the right to ask that your name be withheld from your employer. OSHA must tell you whether or not an inspection will be performed in response to your complaint and the reasons for the decision.

For more information consult OSHA's web page on how to file a complaint: http://www.osha.gov/as/opa/worker/complaint.html

---

Checklist for Nurses

Use this checklist to keep track of the progress that you and your colleagues make in reducing, controlling, and eliminating the safety and health hazards in your workplace.

❑ Contact your state nurses' association (SNA) for information, resources and support.

❑ Learn about the safety and health hazards that may exist in your facility.

❑ Assess the need for workplace hazard control measures.

❑ Teach your colleagues about the importance of documenting illnesses and injuries.

❑ Know your rights in the workplace.

❑ Request and become familiar with the OSHA standards that apply to your workplace.

❑ Request information from your facility and/or NIOSH regarding the chemicals used.

❑ Analyze Material Safety Data Sheets (MSDSs).

❑ Request access to exposure, medical, group and workers' compensation data and records.

❑ Review your workplace OSHA 200 log.

❑ Establish a health and safety committee *or* ensure that an RN is on an existing committee.

❑ Conduct a workplace walk-through.

❑ Seek assistance from government agencies and resources as needed.

❑ File a complaint with OSHA.

❑ Request that OSHA inspect your work site.

❑ Request a NIOSH Health Hazard Evaluation (HHE).

❑ File workers' compensation claims when appropriate.

❑ Contact your local-area Committee for Occupational Safety and Health (COSH). COSH groups are organizations of health and safety advocates. Consult Appendix J to find the address and telephone number of your local COSH group

2

USING THE OSHA 200 LOG
AND OTHER SOURCES

Can restructuring be hazardous to your health? Are you and your colleagues caring for more patients with fewer RNs? Have you strained your back or neck while moving a patient? Nurses in Minnesota suspected that more and more of their colleagues were suffering from occupational illnesses and injuries, while at the same time many Minnesota facilities were downsizing their nursing staff. But what could they do? There were no studies on this issue, no "evidence." So, the Minnesota Nurses Association (MNA) decided to work with their members to prove what they intuitively knew was happening in their state.

MNA requested and received OSHA 200 logs from 12 hospitals covering a four-year period. They analyzed the data and discovered a disturbing 65.2 percent increase in the number of occupational injuries and illnesses among RNs from 1990 to 1994. During that same time period, RN positions had been reduced by 9.2 percent.

In the previous chapter, you learned about your rights under the OSH Act and other resources available to assure your right to a "safe and healthful workplace". This chapter will discuss how to use the OSHA 200 log to gather information about the occupational injuries and illnesses in your facility. You will learn how to analyze the information from the log for use as evidence of health and safety problems in your facility.

You can submit this research to OSHA and other federal agencies when you file a complaint. Just as the MNA nurses did, you can work with your SNA to study and analyze the OSHA 200 logs from your facility to determine whether your employer is meeting its legal obligation to provide a "safe and healthful workplace".

The OSHA 200 Log

This section details use of the OSHA Form No. 200, Log and Summary of Occupational Injuries and Illnesses, commonly known as the OSHA 200 Log.

What Records Are Kept on Occupational Injuries and Illnesses?

The Occupational Safety and Health (OSH) Act of 1970 requires most employers (private-sector employers with 11 or more employees) to prepare and maintain records of occupational injuries and illnesses (see title 29, Code of Federal Regulations, part 1904). Those records include OSHA Form No. 200, Log and Summary of Occupational Injuries and Illnesses, and OSHA Form No. 101, Supplementary Record of Occupational Injuries and Illnesses.

OSHA, part of the U.S. Department of Labor, enforces the record-keeping standard. The Bureau of Labor Statistics (BLS) administers the record-keeping system. OSHA and BLS use the data collected from OSHA Form No. 200 and OSHA Form No. 101 in several ways.

OSHA uses the data to determine rates of injury or illness and lost workdays, to assess the effectiveness of safety and health programs, and to target areas for inspections. BLS compiles and categorizes injuries and fatalities by Standard Industrial Classification (SIC) code and publishes the information for public use. Visit www.bls.gov or call 1-202-606-5886 for a listing of SIC publications.

What Is the OSHA 200 Log?

OSHA Form No. 200, Log and Summary of Occupational Injuries and Illnesses, is commonly known as the OSHA 200 Log. It is used to record and classify all recordable occupational injuries and illnesses. Work-related fatalities and catastrophic events that result in the hospitalization of three or more employees also must be recorded and reported to OSHA within eight hours.

Note: Beginning January 1, 2002, OSHA's new recordkeeping rule, which was issued on January 19, 2001 as a revision of their old recordkeeping rule (29 CFR 1904), will be enforced. Under the new rule, employers will be required to record and keep work-related injury and illness information on an OSHA 300 Log, whose use will become effective January 1, 2002. (A comparison of the OSHA 200 and 300 Logs is in Appendix N along with a copy of the new OSHA 300 Log.)

OSHA defines recordable occupational injuries and illnesses as those involving loss of consciousness, restriction of work or motion, transfer to another job, or medical treatment other than first aid. Your employer must record the following information for each work-related injury or illness that occurs during the calendar year:

■ case or file number that corresponds to the number on the supplementary OSHA Form No. 101;

■ date of injury;

■ employee name;

■ employee occupation;

■ department where the employee regularly works (whether or not that department is where the injury or illness occurred);

■ description of injury or illness;

- date of fatality, if injury-related;

- extent and outcome of injury, including number of days away from work or with restricted work activity; and

- type, extent of, and outcome of illness, including number of days away from work or with restricted work activity.

Besides recording descriptive information in the log, your employer uses a checklist to maintain a running total of the number of injuries and illnesses, and related time away from work or time performing restricted work for each injury or illness.

Your employer also must complete an OSHA Form No. 101, Supplementary Record of Occupational Injuries and Illnesses, for each injury, illness, or fatality recorded on the OSHA 200 Log. See Appendix K for a copy of OSHA Form No. 101.

How Can I Use the OSHA 200 Log?

The OSHA 200 Log can be a valuable tool that you can use to:

- ensure that your employer is accurately addressing safety and health issues,

- determine whether your employer is meeting the legal obligation to provide a safe and healthful workplace,

- find out where most of the injuries and illnesses are occurring, and

- identify what types of injuries occur the most frequently.

With this information, you can decide what types of changes need to be made and where. Safety and health committees can use log information to target unsafe work areas and to work for better conditions.

Additionally, your safety and health committee can double-check OSHA 200 Logs for accuracy and completeness by keeping its own records on injuries and illnesses that occur in your workplace. If you suspect that your employer is falsifying or failing to maintain records, you should file an OSHA complaint. See Chapter 1 or refer to OSHA 29 CFR 1904.

A Closer Look at the OSHA 200 Log

The OSHA 200 Log can be intimidating, but it is a valuable source of information and is less complex than a patient's chart. Use this overview to help you understand what information is kept in the OSHA 200 Log and how to analyze it. OSHA Log 200 is reproduced on the next two pages. (*Note:* Please also refer to Appendix N for a comparison of the OSHA 200 and 300 Logs. The latter form will be effective as of January 1, 2002.)

Columns A–F, the first six columns, on the OSHA 200 Log provide information related to the injury or illness. When looking at those columns, ask the following questions. (*Note:* Since the columns are designated differently on the OSHA 200 and 300 Logs, each form's column is identified.)

- When did the injury or onset of illness occur? (OSHA 200, B; OSHA 300, D)

- Who is being injured or becoming ill? (OSHA 200, C; OSHA 300, B)

- Are the injuries and illnesses occurring in isolated cases or in groups of employees? (OSHA 200, D and E; OSHA 300, C and E)

Log and Summary of Occupational Injuries and Illnesses

NOTE: This form is required by Public Law 91-596 and must be kept in the establishment for 5 years. Failure to maintain and post can result in issuance of citations and assessment of penalties.

(See posting requirements on the other side of form)

RECORDABLE CASES: You are required to record information about every occupational death; every nonfatal occupational illness; and those nonfatal occupational injuries which involve one or more of the following: loss of conciousness, restriction of work or motion, transfer to another job, or medical treatment (other than first aid)

(See definitions on the other side of form)

(A) Case or File Number	(B) Date of Injury or Onset of Illness	(C) Employee's Name	(D) Occupation	(E) Department	(F) Description of Injury or Illness
Enter a nonduplicating number which will facilitate comparisons with supplementary records.	Enter Mo/Day	Enter first name or initial, middle initial, last name	Enter regular job title, not activity employee was performing when injury occurred or at onset of illness. In the absence of a formal title, enter a brief description of the employee's duties.	Enter department in which the employee is regularly employed or a description of normal workplace to which employee is assigned, even though temporarily working in another department at the time of injury or illness.	Enter a brief description of the injury or illness and indicate the part or parts of the body affected. Typical entries for this column might be: Amputation of 1st joint right forefinger; Strain of lower back; Contact dermatitis on both hands; Electrocution - body.
					PREVIOUS PAGE TOTALS =>
					TOTALS (Instructions on other side of form) =>

OSHA No. 200

U.S. Department of Labor

For Calendar Year _____

Page: _____ of _____

Form Approved
O.M.B. No. 1218-0176
See OMB Disclosure
Statement on reverse.

Company Name _____
Establishment Name _____
Establishment Address _____

Extent of and Outcome of Injury

Fatalities

(1) Injury Related — Enter Date of death. mm/dd/yy

Nonfatal Injuries

Injuries with Lost Workdays

- (2) Enter a Check if injury involves DAYS away from work or restricted work activity or both.
- (3) Enter number of DAYS away from work.
- (4) Enter number of DAYS of restricted work activity
- (5) Enter number of DAYS of restricted work activity

Injuries Without Lost Workdays

- (6) Enter a Check if no entry was made in column 1 or 2 but the injury is recordable as defined above.

Type, Extent of, and Outcome of Illness

Type of Illness

(7) CHECK Only One Column for Each Illness (See other side of form for terminations or permanent transfers)

- (a) Occupational Skin Disorder or Disease
- (b) Dust Disease of the lungs
- (c) Respiratory Conditions due to toxic agents
- (d) Poisoning (systemic effects of toxic materials)
- (e) Disorders due to physical agents
- (f) Disorders associated with repeated trauma
- (g) All other occupational illnesses

Fatalities

(8) Illness Related — Enter DATE of death, mm/dd/yy

Nonfatal Illnesses

Illnesses with Lost Workdays

- (9) Enter a CHECK if Illness involves DAYS away from work, or DAYS of restricted work activity or both.
- (10) Enter a CHECK if Illness involves DAYS away from work.
- (11) Enter number of DAYS away from work.
- (12) Enter number of DAYS of restricted work activity

Illnesses without Lost Workdays

- (13) Enter a CHECK if no entry was made in columns 8 or 9

Certification of Annual Summary Totals by: _____   Title: _____   Date: _____

POST ONLY THIS PORTION OF THE LAST PAGE NO LATER THAN FEBRUARY 1

OSHA 200

■ Are the injuries and illnesses happening to employees in some job titles and not others? (OSHA 200, D; OSHA 300, E)

■ Where are the injuries occurring and which departments have more injuries or illnesses? (OSHA 200, E; OSHA 300, F)

■ Do certain types of injury or illness outnumber others? (OSHA 200, F and columns 7a–g; OSHA 300, 1–7)

Compare the types of injuries and illnesses by department and by job title. By noting similarities and differences, you can locate areas in your workplace that have possible safety and health concerns. Examples might include employees who have not been given adequate safety and health training, personal protective equipment, recent equipment changes, adequate staffing levels, or safe areas to work in.

Columns 1–6 and columns 8–13 provide information on the severity or seriousness of the injury (1-6) or illness (8-13), characterized by whether or not the employee, as a result of the injury or illness, was absent from work or worked with restricted duties. (In the OSHA 300 Log, columns H, I, K, and L.)

In looking at those columns, compare the description of the injury or illness in column F (in both forms 200 and 300) with the number of absent or restricted duty days. You should see a connection between the type of injury and the number of days. If they do not seem to correspond, perhaps the employee used vacation or sick time instead, and thus the days were not counted as work-related absences.

Do you know any co-workers who continue to perform their regular job duties despite health care providers asking them to restrict their duties? How many of you do whatever it takes to get the job done, regardless of the personal health consequences? The OSHA 200 Log does not capture those instances. Remember, the log is only as useful as the accuracy of its recorded information. *Educate your colleagues to report all job-associated injuries and illnesses to the occupational health department and to request that these incidents be recorded in the OSHA 200 Log.*

Columns 7a–g describe the illness shown in column 7. Where are certain types of illnesses categorized? If the employee becomes ill following the needlestick injury, the incident would be placed in column 7g (M-7 in OSHA 300), All Other Occupational Illnesses, which would include Hepatitis B, C, D, and E; HIV; and all other bloodborne diseases. However, if no illness occurred as a result of the stick, the incident may be checked under an injury column 6 (J in OSHA 300), but no illness column would be checked. Thus, when counting injuries and illnesses due to needlestick injuries, you might have to look under both the injury and illness categories. Unfortunately, because column 7g includes other illnesses besides bloodborne diseases, you will need to closely compare the illness type with the description in column F.

What are the illness categories for latex allergy? They may be listed under column 7a (M-3 in OSHA 300), Occupational Skin Diseases or Disorders, for dermatitis reactions. They also may be listed under column 7e, Disorders Due to Physical Agents, for conditions such as occupational asthma or respiratory conditions due to toxic agents.

Which column contains checks for musculoskeletal disorders such as carpal tunnel syndrome, tendinitis, and Raynaud's syndrome? You would look in column 7f, Disorders Associated with Repeated Traumas (M-2, Musculoskeletal Disorders, in OSHA 300), and in the injury columns for acute musculoskeletal disorders such as back, neck, or shoulder strains.

By counting the number in each category of injury or illness, you can compare that amount with totals for different years, departments, and job titles. That information can help you to identify areas where safety and health problems exist.

Applying Epidemiological Analysis to OSHA 200 Log Data

Epidemiological data analysis from the OSHA 200 Log provides methods for looking at causes of disease or injury occurring in groups of people. Taking an epidemiological approach, you can:

- examine causes of injuries and illnesses,
- identify high-risk work,
- determine why certain groups of workers have injuries or illness and other workers do not,
- evaluate safety and health program effectiveness (such as training, personal protective equipment, and engineering controls), and
- provide data to use in developing safety and health control measures.

Epidemiology allows you to count the number of injuries or illnesses and related lost workdays found in the OSHA 200 Log for your workplace in a given year. You then can compare those numbers with other years at your workplace, with other workplaces, or with national data for your type of workplace. Such comparisons can help you to assess whether the number and severity of occupational injuries and illnesses is better or worse than expected for your type of workplace and whether they are increasing or decreasing over time. The following paragraphs discuss several types of epidemiology methods, such as counts, ratios, and rates.

Counts

Counts of injuries, illnesses, or any other data from the OSHA 200 Log provide information that characterizes a group of employees' injury and illness events. The log already provides checks you can count for injuries, illnesses, days away from work, days of restricted work, and fatalities. You can further break down those counts by subcategories, such as the number of one specific type of injury (back strain, for example), the number of days away from work for all types of strain, and so on. You can then compare those counts with other years, other work areas, and the like.

Answer the following questions using the OSHA 200 Log and information about your workplace:

- Which unit in your workplace has the most days away from work? Count the number of checks in columns 4 and 11 (in Form 300, H and number of days in K and L) for each separate department listed in column E (in both Forms 200 and 300) and compare the departments. Are the numbers similar across departments? Are any departments showing much higher counts? The answers can give you an indication of where the greatest amount of time is lost because of injuries or illness at work.

■ What do you know about each department? Are there differences in the types of patient care? Are there differences in staffing levels? Is the type of work different in the department with highest counts versus the department with the lowest count? Are there unique safety and health hazards in some departments and not in others? The answers can help you to identify possible safety and health concerns.

■ Count the checks in columns 5 and 12 (I and K in Form 300) and compare the total days of restricted work activity by department for. By identifying the departments with the greatest number of restricted workdays, you can begin to see where the most serious injuries and illnesses occur in your workplace. Conversely, by counting the number of injuries and illnesses without lost workdays (in columns 6 and 13; I and J in Form 300)), you can determine the types of injuries and illnesses that were less serious, and where they occurred by identifying the departments listed in column E (in both forms). The results can help you to prioritize areas (job titles and departments) that most require better safety and health prevention measures.

■ Next, count the number of each kind of injury or illness, using both column F (in both forms) and columns 7a–g (M-1 through M-7 in OSHA 300). Are similar kinds of injuries or illnesses occurring in all departments, or do certain departments have greater numbers of a certain type of injury or illness? Do some job titles have greater numbers of some injuries or illnesses than other job titles? What is similar and different among the various departments which you are comparing? What is similar and different about the types of jobs done by the injured or ill employees? The answers can help you identify departments and jobs that may have a higher risk of injury or illness.

Once you identify the departments and jobs with higher or lower numbers of injuries and illnesses, you can ask more questions to help determine what safety and health problems may exist:

■ Are there specific safety and health problems that are widespread in your workplace? You most likely would count similar numbers of injuries (for example, needlesticks) and illnesses for multiple departments (for example, all nursing units) if that were true.

■ Are the safety and health problems limited to some departments? That would be evident if, for instance, the greatest number of back injuries were in the orthopedic and head injury units. You can then begin to identify the causes of work-related injuries and illnesses.

■ How many illnesses are there in column 7d (M-5 in OSHA 300) for this year compared with last year's OSHA 200 Log? The answer can help you determine whether safety and health prevention measures are working in your workplace. An increase in numbers can be a clue that prevention measures are inadequate. Do counts and comparisons for column F (in both forms) and columns 7a–g (M-2 through M-7 in OSHA 300).

■ Do some employee names appear several times for injuries or illnesses? Count the number of times each employee has been injured or become ill.

■ Are their injuries similar each time? If yes, you might infer that some employees require specific types of training that may be lacking.

■ What do you know about those employees? Are they new to your workplace, their department, or their job title? If so, perhaps they were improperly trained, assigned heavy loads or are not aware of lifting or needle devices that prevent injuries.

■ Are any injury- or illness-related deaths marked in column 1 or column 8? If so, what is the description of the injury or illness in column F, the department in column E, and the job title in column D? The answers can provide clues to hazardous work or work areas in your workplace that can be lethal.

Rates and Ratios

Rates and ratios are methods of comparing one count with another. For example, you might compare the number of one type of injury with the number of another type of injury, or you might compare the number of injured or ill employees with the number of all employees working at a specified time. Rates and ratios take one count and divide it by another. The resulting number can be shown as a percentage or proportion.

Severity rates measure the seriousness of conditions by lost work days (columns 3 and 10) or days with restricted work activities (columns 4 and 11). You can also look at the number of those days combined (columns 2 and 9). Additionally, ratios and rates can be calculated for injuries and illnesses, injuries only, illnesses only, fatalities only, lost workday cases, nonfatal cases without lost workdays, or number of lost workdays.

Answer the following questions using the OSHA 200 Log and information about your workplace to determine rates and ratios of injuries and illnesses:

■ *What proportion of disorders associated with repeated trauma resulted in lost or restricted workdays?* Divide the total number of disorders—those associated with illnesses and repeated trauma that result in lost or restricted workdays— in column 9 by the total number of disorders associated with repeated trauma in column 7f. The result of your calculation is a percentage that tells you the proportion of disorders associated with repeated trauma that required time away from work or restricted work duty. You can then compare that number with similar calculations from previous years of OSHA 200 Logs to see whether the percentage has gone up or down. An increase would indicate a need for stronger safety and health prevention methods.

■ *What proportion of disorders associated with repeated trauma had no time away from work?* Divide the total number of disorders without lost workdays in column 13 by the total number of disorders associated with repeated trauma in column 7f. The result of your calculation is a percentage that tells you the proportion of disorders associated with repeated trauma that had no time away from work. Again, you can compare that number with previous years.

■ *How do the percentages for disorders associated with repeated trauma that resulted in lost or restricted workdays compare with those that required no time away from work?* Safety and health prevention aimed at decreasing the cases of the most severe disorders associated with repeated trauma would focus on the departments and job titles associated with lost or restricted workdays. This is another way of prioritizing severity and relating it to the department or job title where the injury or illness resulted in the greatest loss of work time.

■ *What proportion of RNs had occupational skin diseases or disorders?* Count the number of checks in column 7a that correspond to the job title of RN in column D. Divide that number by the total number of RNs employed at your workplace. The number you end up with is the percentage of RNs who had occupational skin diseases or disorders during the calendar year.

■ Repeat your calculations for each job title (column D) or department (column E) and the various injuries or illnesses (column F and columns 7a–g). The results can help you determine whether certain injuries or illnesses represent a large proportion of the entire number of employees in each job title or department. The ones with larger proportions represent areas to investigate for safety and health issues that need improvement.

Incidence and prevalence rates and other rate calculations are used by various agencies (for example, the Bureau of Labor Statistics, the National Safety Council, and OSHA) or safety and health personnel (for example, the human resources and employee safety and health departments).

Incidence rates show the extent or frequency of new injuries or illnesses in a specific group of employees (such as your hospital) during a specified period of time (such as a year). Prevalence rates measure the total numbers of injuries or illnesses that exist in a group of employees at a given time. You can use incidence and prevalence rates to suggest the likelihood of risk and to study the etiology of an injury or illness. However, the calculations for incidence and prevalence are complicated and may be less useful for your purposes.

Principles to Keep in Mind

Epidemiological methods give you tools that can help you to make sense of the OSHA 200 Log. However, the information that you produce must be used within the context of your workplace. Look at the counts of injuries or illnesses in relation to the affected employees, the job titles, the departments, and the timing of the injuries or illnesses. If you work in a merged institution, compare the information that you find from your workplace with that in your sister hospital.

Finally, answer the following questions for clues to the causes of injuries and illnesses and for potential prevention measures that can be taken in response to them:

■ You have counted the injuries or illnesses and discover that they have occurred over a certain period or only in a certain department. What was happening, or not happening, in that department or during that period? The answer can give you clues to safety and health concerns.

- What do you think may have been the cause? To answer this question, look at the staffing and acuity levels for the period that you are examining. Was work redesigned or were new work practices implemented? Were any of the injured or ill employees newly hired?

- How much time elapsed between possible causes (risks or hazards) and the injuries or illnesses?

Other Information Sources

Not all of the answers to your safety and health related questions can be found in the OSHA 200 Log. There are other sources of information within and outside your workplace.

Information Sources in Your Workplace

The following sources of information from within your workplace may be available to you.

- Accident investigation forms.

- Safety and health committee minutes documenting discussions of accidents and incidents.

- Assignment Despite Objection forms.

- Absenteeism data, and other employee records.

- Accounts from your fellow employees.

Assignment Despite Objection Forms

Assignment Despite Objection (ADO) forms were developed by state nurses' associations to document unsafe staffing and professional concerns. These forms include a space for objecting to the assignment because it poses a serious health and safety threat. Contact your state nurses' association for information on how best to use the ADO forms.

Absenteeism and Other Employee Records

Records of high absenteeism in certain departments of your workplace may indicate problems related to safety and health. As a result, you may find it useful to compare lost workdays from the OSHA 200 Log with records for sick and vacation leave to determine whether employees are using personal time for work-related injuries rather than using the workers' compensation system.

Other safety and health-related records—such as short-term and long-term disability information, accommodation information under the Americans with Disabilities Act (ADA), accident investigations, etc.—may be kept at your workplace. Such information can shed light on areas with safety and health problems that have not been recorded on the OSHA 200 Log.

This kind of information is *not* accessible to you by law. However, personnel from your human resources, risk management, or safety and health departments may be willing to share group data, if individual employees are not identified. If your workplace has an employee health nurse or an occupational health nurse, he or she can help you to determine what additional records you might want to request, and how to use those records to identify safety and health priorities in your work area. Although all of these people work for your employer, they can become great allies to you. Learn who they are and what their safety and health roles are in your workplace.

Assistance and Sources of Information Outside Your Workplace

Contact your state nurses' association for information or assistance with any of these sources.

■ OSHA web site and Expert Advisor software programs.

■ Bureau of Labor Statistics (BLS) yearly injury and illness data, reported by Standard Industrial Classification (SIC) code.

■ Workers' compensation statistics (your own or data on groups of employees).

■ Centers for Disease Control and Prevention (CDC).

■ National Safety Council (NSC).

■ Internet access to agencies, libraries and associations that keep updated information, references, and contact numbers.

OSHA Web Site and Expert Advisor Software Programs

Visit OSHA's web site (www.osha.gov) to review OSHA citations by Standard Industrial Classification (SIC) code and region of the country. Enter an SIC code, state, or city to narrow your search on the OSHA web site.

The U.S. Government's SIC Manual classifies businesses by the type of activity in which they are engaged, using a hierarchical coding system. For example, in this system:

■ the SIC code for all health services is 80;

■ the code for nursing homes, known as "nursing and personal care facilities," is 805;

■ hospitals are classified in SIC code 806; and

■ home health care has SIC code 808.

OSHA Expert Advisor software programs are computerized "expert systems" which enable businesses and others to answer a few simple questions and receive reliable answers on how OSHA regulations apply to their unique work sites. Expert Advisor programs are provided free and can be downloaded and run on local personal computers. The Expert Advisors combine the expertise of OSHA safety and health professionals, including epidemiologists, risk assessors, and attorneys, into a single source of expert help. Go to http://www.osha-slc.gov/dts/osta/oshasoft/ for a menu of the available Expert Advisors.

Bureau of Labor Statistics Data

In recent years, federal agencies have started paying attention to the growing dangers of working in the health care environment. The latest Bureau of Labor

Statistics (BLS) data indicate an increase in the rates of injuries and illnesses for healthcare workers, while the average rate for workers in private industries continues to fall. In terms of lost workdays as a result of work-related injury, it is now more dangerous to work in a nursing home than it is to work in the mining or construction industry.

BLS annually reports safety and health statistics by Standard Industrial Classification (SIC) codes in *Compensation and Working Conditions Safety and Health Statistics.* By determining the SIC code for your workplace, you can compare the data which you have collected on injuries and illnesses in your workplace with similar places of employment.

Workers' Compensation Data

Workers' compensation is a no-fault insurance system that provides partial wage replacement and medical payments if you are injured on the job or contract a work-related illness.

Each state has its own workers' compensation program, and the programs differ considerably in terms of the adequacy of benefits, costs, coverage, and efficiency of administration. Check with your state workers' compensation board for information related to data collected on occupational injuries and illnesses of interest to your workplace.

In addition, group data for injuries and illnesses covered under workers' compensation will be available in varying degrees according to state and federal privacy laws, such as state freedom of information acts.

You also may be able to obtain workers' compensation data from your own workplace. Various departments—such as human resources, personnel,, or risk management—or the employee health nurse may keep internal records related to types of claims and costs related to those claims.

While the OSH Act does not require your employer to share *group* workers' compensation data with employees, you can request access to your *own* workers' compensation file. You should make your request in writing.

Not all injuries and illnesses on the OSHA 200 Log become workers' compensation claims. Some are not serious enough to require a claim. Others are not documented under workers' compensation because employees choose to see their own private physicians, pay for the visits with group medical insurance, and, if any absences from work are required, use their personal sick or vacation leave. *Again, all systems of tracking are only as useful as the information recorded, so encourage your colleagues to report and document **all** work-related injuries and illnesses.*

Centers for Disease Control and Prevention Data

The Centers for Disease Control and Prevention (CDC) collect data on communicable diseases, such as tuberculosis and hepatitis, and publish them in a weekly document called the *Morbidity and Mortality Weekly Report,* or *MMWR.* Your employer can subscribe to the *MMWR* through its library or the employee safety and health department.

You can find the *MMWR* and guidelines for safe work practices related to blood-borne pathogens on CDC's web site at www.cdc.gov, or through ANA's web site at www.nursingworld.org/dlwa/osh/ .

National Safety Council Data

The National Safety Council publishes *Accident Facts*, a yearly statistical report on accidental deaths, injuries, and related costs. It provides data on work accidents by type of injury, costs, and workers' compensation reports. It also includes BLS incidence rates. A small section is devoted to occupational illnesses. For more information about *Accident Facts*, call the National Safety Council's toll-free number at 1-800-621-7619.

Counting Costs

Counting costs can help you to demonstrate to management how expensive occupational injuries and illnesses really are, and how the employer can save money by improving safety and health in your workplace.

When figuring the costs of an injury or illness, you should add in both the direct and indirect costs. The direct costs of an injury or illness include:

- medical payments to health care providers,

- lost-wage payments,

- costs for replacing staff who cannot work,

- administrative costs for workers' compensation claims, and

- post-exposure testing and prophylactic medications.

Indirect costs are those related to the lost productivity and decreased quality of services that occur when valued employees are off work or unable to fully perform their duties.

While you may not have access to all direct and indirect cost data, you can estimate overall costs for an injury or illness by using what you do have available. For example, you can estimate medical payments by contacting an insurance company and requesting reimbursement rates for certain types of health care provider visits. Then, you can estimate indirect costs at two to fifty times the direct costs. You can determine the cost of lost productivity and decreased quality of services by multiplying the hourly rates of injured/ill workers times the number of days away from work. The following example shows how to count costs related to a hypothetical injury:

What can you do with this information? You can show your employer that it is far less expensive to buy a patient lift device and train nurses to use it than it is to pay for even one back injury. To illustrate, assume that the lift costs $6,000 and the training costs $750 (wages for 15 nurses at $25/hour for 2 hours). Together, these two preventive measures total $6,750, which is in the range of the above estimates for just one injury. You can use the same process of counting costs to show the benefit of adding staff, as well as purchasing equipment. (See the next page for these calculations.)

RN with a Back Strain

Direct costs:

3 physician or nurse practitioner visits × $60 = $180

5 days off work × $200/day = $1,000

5 days of replacement staff × $300/day = $1,500

3 hours for claim administration × $15/hour = $45

Total direct costs = $2,725

Indirect costs estimated two ways:

(1) Wages of RN ($200/day) × 5 days = $1,000

(2) Total direct costs ($2,725) × 2 = $5,450

Total costs are estimated between $3,725 and $8,175. Both are conservative estimates.

3

PROMOTING HEALTH AND SAFETY AT YOUR FACILITY

The Occupational Safety and Health Act alone does not provide comprehensive protection to nurses and other health care workers. Without a complaint being filed, OSHA is able to randomly inspect covered workplaces only once every 75 years. In addition, not all workplaces are covered by OSHA. Public employees in many states are still without federal health and safety protections.

Due to the slow and contentious regulatory process, OSHA has not yet published standards on many serious hazards faced by health care workers (i.e., tuberculosis [TB] and violence). Surprisingly, exposure limits have not been established for most of the toxic chemicals used. Although many health care employers insist that letter-of-the-law compliance with existing regulations is adequate, this level of protection is unsafe and far less than nurses deserve.

The benchmarking process—that is, assessing the "community standards and guidelines" being used throughout the industry and coming in line with those practices—is widely used in the health care industry to improve patient care delivery. This benchmarking process is equally applicable to improving health and safety for workers. Nurses, with their strong assessment and problem-solving skills, are necessary participants in this process.

First Steps

■ Join a health and safety committee. It is essential that nursing be a part of this committee. OSHA has a Safety and Health Programs Advisor that can help you <http://www.osha-slc.gov/dts/osta/oshasoft>

■ Educate yourself and your colleagues. Health and safety programs require a foundation of knowledge about the issues and an awareness of the relationship between health and safety and workplace rights.

■ Collect data. Several different systems exist to track health and safety data in hospitals. Each system reveals slightly different information.

■ Identify and review current health and safety policies. More regulatory agencies are checking to see that polices actually reflect reality at a particular workplace and that the latest knowledge and standards are incorporated.

■ Identify and review the Material Safety Data Sheets (MSDSs) for all hazardous chemicals and drugs used in the workplace.

■ Don't forget to include the use and review of Assignment Despite Objection forms to see if there is pattern of injuries and illnesses among nurses linked to periods of inadequate staffing.

Assessing Current Efforts

The Joint Commission on the Accreditation of Health Care Facilities Organizations (JCAHO), with its mission of protecting patient care safety, requires that inpatient facilities establish a safety committee that meets at least six times per year. The structure of this committee should allow for representation from workers and managers alike, with equal input and control of the agenda. JCAHO's Environment of Care guidelines often dictate core activities committee, but the committee should be open to addressing any health and safety issues identified. It is essential that nursing staff be an integral part of this team. If possible, a nurse representative from the safety committee should also sit on the hospital's new product or purchasing committee to screen for products that may adversely affect worker health and safety.

During JCAHO visits, inspectors look for documentation proving that a system is in place to address hazards, and that the hazards reported are addressed. JCAHO has very few specific health and safety requirements that apply solely to worker health and safety. However, the emphasis on a safe environment of care for patients can also improve conditions for workers.

Collecting Data

In the previous chapter, you learned how to collect and analyze data. One of the many reasons to "document, document, document" is to have the data to demonstrate that a problem exists. A health and safety committee should regularly review and analyze data from the following sources:

■ OSHA Logs of Employee Injury and Illness

■ Detailed reports of exposures to bloodborne pathogens, including devices causing the injuries and seroconversions

■ Infections control reports of disease transmission related to the environment or workers

■ Reports of TB exposure follow-up and PPD skin testing program effectiveness

■ Security reports, especially reports of threats and assaults

■ Fire safety incidents and outcomes

■ Records of scheduled workplace walkthroughs, audits, and inspections

■ Patient and employee incident reports

- Mechanical and utility incident reports
- Logs of student and volunteer injury and illness
- Biomechanical engineering records of defective equipment
- Records of compliance with annual health and safety training and education

Nurses may also want to suggest that the committee review Assignment Despite Objection forms or Protest of Assignment forms in relation to possible increases in occurrences of injury and illness among nurses at those times.

Reviewing Health and Safety Policies

Policy work is sometimes viewed by nurses as a "paper-only" exercise that does little to affect real life. It becomes relevant only if integrated into day-to-day nursing practice.

Developing health and safety policies means that you approach health and safety hazards with the big picture in mind. This is a "system-fix" approach, a method recently advocated by the prestigious Institute of Medicine as a means to reduce health care errors. This approach, along with the goal of establishing an open, non-judgmental environment for reporting incidents and near-misses, is the hallmark of innovative error and accident prevention.

To develop, revise, and update policies, the latest standards, guidelines, and peer-reviewed studies should be gathered. New strategies should be presented and discussed in the safety committee, keeping in mind the goals: hazard reduction and worker injury and illness prevention. Buy-in from unit managers should be sought for anticipated changes to their policies and areas. Most important, ultimate decision-makers should be educated about the subject prior to being pressed for a decision.

The bottom line is the act of integrating policies in everyday practice through effective training and education. If this step doesn't occur, then health and safety policy work *is* a paper exercise.

Improving the Effectiveness of Health and Safety Prevention Efforts

"Evidence-based" practice, aimed at improving clinical treatment effectiveness, is not limited to the care of patients. Health and safety professionals must also rely on the body of literature in their field to identify the most effective prevention measures to protect workers. The pace of federal health and safety regulation lags far behind that of medical and scientific publications. Because of this, whoever is involved in developing or revising health and safety policies must also consider the evidence in the peer-reviewed literature, alerts and guidelines from government agencies, and recommendations from professional organizations. Important resources for the major hazards are discussed below. Many other useful publications are listed in Appendix M, Additional Web Resources.

HIV, Hepatitis, and Other Bloodborne Pathogens

The responsibilities of health care employers in preventing bloodborne disease transmission to workers are clearly outlined by the OSHA Bloodborne Pathogens Standard. Few other hazards are as thoroughly regulated. It is because of this standard that we've witnessed the dramatic decline of occupational infection with Heptitis B, since the standard required employers to provide Hepatitis B vaccine to workers at risk of exposure.

Within the standard, OSHA refers to the most current guidelines from the Centers for Disease Control and Prevention (CDC) for the treatment and follow-up of workers who sustain a bloodborne pathogens exposure. These "post-exposure prophylaxis" guidelines are organized by pathogen (HIV, Heptitis C, Hepatitis B) and are updated as the newest treatment options become available. Your hospital employee health unit and safety committee should be providing treatment according to these latest guidelines, readily available from the CDC.

Due to the success of ANA's Safe Needles Save Lives Campaign, the OSHA Bloodborne Pathogens Standard was recently amended. Now health care employers are required to provide safety devices that more effectively prevent needlestick and sharp exposures. There are also new requirements for documenting the circumstances surrounding the exposure, especially the name and brand of the device causing exposure.

Tuberculosis

For nearly 10 years, health care workers have sought, and OSHA has attempted to finalize, a standard to prevent occupational transmission of TB. However, the health care industry and some professional organizations would prefer to see TB prevention measures remain voluntary. Currently, standard health and safety practice is based on the CDC's current recommendations for the prevention of TB in healthcare facilities; however, there is considerable debate about the effectiveness of these guidelines because of their voluntary nature. Check the OSHA and CDC websites for the latest progress on TB standards and guidelines.

One of the biggest controversies in this hazard area has been over the appropriate respiratory protection needed to prevent workers' exposure to TB. Although OSHA can cite employers for not providing the correct type of respirators, the National Institute for Occupational Safety and Health (NIOSH) is actually the agency responsible for approving the types and brands of respirators that can be used. Helpful resources are available from these two organizations. See Appendix H and Appendix M.

Latex Allergy

In the early 1990s, nurses and affected patient groups alerted the country to the hazards associated with latex, namely, allergic reactions. Through letters, testimony at federal agencies, and case reports, the nursing and health care worker communities were able to focus the attention of allergy and immunology researchers on the problem. Although the body of literature has grown tremendously in the last 10 years, OSHA has not yet agreed to begin work on a standard. Instead, the agency placed the issue on their "non-regulatory calendar" and the Office of Occupational Medicine issued a voluntary technical information bulletin.

The most important document influencing the course of latex allergy prevention efforts was the 1997 NIOSH alert entitled "Preventing Allergic Reactions to Latex in the Workplace." It strongly recommended the use of powder-free, non-latex gloves in place of traditional powdered latex gloves and amelioration of dust-borne latex proteins, which may trigger allergic reactions. Adherence to NIOSH recommendations is also voluntary.

Because gloves are a medical product, the Food and Drug Administration (FDA) is responsible for regulations governing glove safety. The agency has stepped cautiously but now has a helpful medical glove guide available through the Center for Devices and Radiologic Health. Many of the FDA regulations are based on technical recommendations from the American Society for Testing and Materials (ASTM), whose technical committees are composed of government and industry scientists. The ASTM develops testing methods that FDA often adopts. The occupational health and infection control communities are eagerly awaiting improved glove selection guidance from the CDC to understand the level of glove protection necessary to protect workers during various medical procedures.

In health care facilities, latex allergy policy development can be complex, involving both worker and patient considerations. A nursing voice is critical. Current resources on latex allergy, along with model policies from other employers, must be individually gathered and evaluated.

Back Injuries and Other Musculoskeletal Disorders (Ergonomics Standard)

Advocates for worker health and safety spent the better part of the decade assuring that an OSHA standard on ergonomics (the science of designing the job to fit the worker) would become a reality. In the last days of the Clinton administration, the final standard was published and became effective early the next year. The standard faced considerable opposition from industry and the Republican congress. In March of 2001, a never-used law known as the Congressional Review Act was used by Congress and the new President to nullify the OSHA Ergonomics Standard. Implementation of the standard was halted by this action, and OSHA is barred from working on a similar standard unless new legislation directing them to do so is passed by both houses of congress and signed by the President.

The Ergonomics Standard was the most important OSHA effort to date in preventing disabling injuries to nurses. In the face of this stinging defeat for nurses and the entire health care worker community, ANA will develop a strong position statement that incorporates the injury prevention principles advocated by OSHA. Nurses can take this document to their health and safety committees to advocate for voluntary efforts on the part of employers. Check the Nursing World web site (www.nursingworld.org/dlwa/osh/) for the latest updates.

Violence in the Workplace

No federal standard for prevention of workplace violence exists. After a rash of incidents in the early 1990s that killed, injured, or endangered health care workers, OSHA issued voluntary guidelines for preventing violence to health care and social service workers. Useful surveys and reporting forms are available at the OSHA web site along with the guidelines.

In the mid 1990s, four states passed legislation increasing the penalties for assaults on health care workers and improving violence prevention training and post-assault treatment and services. Check with your local police department about these laws. Victim support services may also have information about your rights if you are assaulted. ANA continues to advocate for improved violence prevention measures for health care workers, preferably an OSHA standard.

Resources from the Nurses at OSHA

The Office of Occupational Health Nursing at OSHA is responsible for some of the most useful documents available on the OSHA web site or through the OSHA Publications Office. At the time this chapter went to press, the nurses at OSHA were working on a guide that should be of great help to those working to promote improved health and safety in their facilities. The title is: "Occupational Safety and Health in the Hospital: A Manual for Hospital Employers."

Moving the Health and Safety Agenda Forward

As RNs, we have to take responsibility for protecting our health and safety. We must take action so that we can care for our patients without jeopardizing our own health. While we face many serious and sometimes deadly hazards, the good news is that we *can* do something about it. We can work with our colleagues and our state nurses' association to take positive steps forward. It is important to share your struggles and successes with your colleagues so we can all benefit from the wisdom of nurses across the nation. As we continue to move the health and safety agenda forward, ANA will continue to be a leader in protecting the health and safety of nurses nationwide.

BIBLIOGRAPHY

Ashford, N.A., and Caldart, C.C. 1991. *Technology, Law and the Working Environment.* New York: Van Nostrand Reinhold.

Brady, W., Bass, J., Moser, R., Anstadt, G.W., Loeppke, R.R., and Leopold, R. 1997. Defining total corporate health and safety costs: significance and impact. *Journal of Occupational and Environmental Medicine* 39(3), 224–231.

Kadish, S., and Weiss, L.D. 1984. *Alaskan Health Hazards in the Workplace: It's Your Right to Know.* Alaska Health Project.

Levy, B.S., and Wegman, D.H., eds. 1995. *Occupational Health: Recognizing and Preventing Work-Related Disease. 3rd ed.* Boston: Little, Brown.

Mausner, J. S., and Kramer, S. 1985. *Epidemiology: An Introductory Text. 2nd ed.* Philadelphia: W.B. Saunders.

National Safety Council. 1990. *Accident Facts.* Chicago: National Safety Council.

Office of the Federal Register. National Archives and Records Administration (1995). Code of Federal Regulations: Labor 29: Parts 1900 to 1910. Washington, D.C.: U.S. Government Printing Office.

State of Washington. Department of Labor and Industries. 1995. *Understanding 'Right to Know': Chemical Hazard Communication Guidelines for Washington Employers.* Olympia.

U.S. Department of Labor. Bureau of Labor Statistics. 1986. *A Brief Guide to Recordkeeping Requirements for Occupational Injuries and Illnesses.* OMB No. 1220-0029. Washington, D.C.: U.S. Government Printing Office.

U.S. Department of Labor. Occupational Safety and Health Administration (OSHA). 1994a. *OSHA: Employee Workplace Rights.* OSHA 3021. Washington, D.C.: U.S. Government Printing Office.

———— 1994b. *Part 1960, Elements for Federal Employee Occupational Safety and Health Programs.* Washington, D.C.: U.S. Government Printing Office.

———— 1993. *Access to Medical and Exposure Records.* OSHA 3110. Washington, D.C.: U.S. Government Printing Office.

———— 1993. *Framework for a Comprehensive Health and Safety Program in the Hospital Environment.* OSHA. Washington, D.C.: U.S. Government Printing Office.

———— 1988. *Recordkeeping and Reporting Guidelines for Federal Agencies.* OSHA 2014. Washington, D.C.: U.S. Government Printing Office.

———— 1986. *Recordkeeping Guidelines for Occupational Injuries and Illnesses.* OMB No. 1220-0029. Washington, D.C.: U.S. Government Printing Office.

APPENDIX A

ANA Occupational/Environmental Health and Safety Resources

Visit ANA's Safety and Health web page at www.nursingworld.org/dlwa/osh/ with links to agencies and organizations protecting health care workers and to articles published in *The American Nurse*. Consult the monthly ANA Health and Safety column in the *American Journal of Nursing*.

Workplace Information Series Brochures

(To order, call ANA Customer Care at 1-800-274-4ANA)

WP-2   HIV, Hepatitis-B, Hepatitis-C Bloodborne Disease

WP-5   Workplace Violence: Can You Close The Door On It?

WP-1   Tuberculosis: A Deadly Disease Makes a Comeback

WP-7   Latex Allergy Protect Yourself Protect Your Patients

EWR12 Passport to Protection Guide to Nurses' Rights (includes a section on OSHA)

ANA Needlestick Prevention Campaign: Safe Needles Save Lives

Visit www.needlestick.org for up-to-date information on needlestick prevention,

Safe Needles Save Lives brochure, stickers and buttons are available from your state nurses association

ANA House of Delegates (HOD) Action Reports on Occupational/Environmental Health

1994   Tuberculosis

1995   Indoor Air Quality

1997   Preventing Health Care Production of Toxic Pollution

1998   Health and Safety Information Report

1999   Safe Needles Save Lives: Preventing Needlestick Injuries (replaces 1991 Position Statement: Availability of Equipment and Safety Procedures to Prevent Transmission of Bloodborne Diseases)

1999   Caring for Those Who Care

ANA Position Statements

1991   Guidelines for Disclosure to a Known Third Party About Possible HIV Infection

1992   HIV Infected Nurse, Ethical Obligations and Disclosure

1994   Risk Versus Responsibility in Providing Nursing Care (This ethics position statement provides the foundation for occupational health and safety provisions in some SNA contracts.)

1997   Latex Allergy

American Nurses Publishing

(To order, call 1-800-637-0323)

NP-82, The Nurse's Shift Work Handbook

EC-151, What You Need to Know about Today's Workplace: A Survival Guide for Nurses

COE-1, What You Need to Know about Today's Workplace: An Independent Study CE Module 9811LA, ANA Pollution Prevention Tool Kit for Nurses

ANA/University of Vermont

Videotape Programs and Independent Study Modules

(To order, call University of Vermont at 1-800-639-3188)

- Natural Rubber Latex Allergy: Recognition, Treatment, and Prevention
- The Healthcare Industry's Impact on the Environment: Strategies for Global Change
- Preventing Needlestick Injuries: The Time Is Now

APPENDIX B

State Nurses Associations Contact Information

For more information, visit ANA's Health and Safety web page at www.nursingworld.org.

Alabama State Nurses Association
360 North Hull Street
Montgomery, Alabama 36104-3658
(334) 262-8321
FAX (334) 262-8578
www.nursingworld.org/snas/al/

Alaska Nurses Association
237 East Third Avenue
Anchorage, Alaska 99501-2523
(907) 274-0827
FAX (907) 272-0292
http://www.aknurse.org

Arizona Nurses Association
1850 E. Southern Ave., Suite #1
Tempe, Arizona 85282
(480) 831-0404
FAX (480) 839-4780
www.nursingworld.org/snas/az

Arkansas Nurses Association
804 N. University
Little Rock, Arkansas 72205
(501) 664-5853
FAX (501) 664-5859
www.arna.org

Colorado Nurses Association
5453 East Evans Place
Denver, Colorado 80222
(303) 757-7483
FAX (303) 757-2679
www.sni.net/cna

Connecticut Nurses Association
Meritech Business Park
377 Research Parkway, Suite 2D
Meriden, Connecticut 06450
(203) 238-1207
FAX (203) 238-3437
www.nursingworld.org/snas/ct

Delaware Nurses Association
2434 Capitol Trail, Suite 330
Newark, Delaware 19711
(302) 368-2333
FAX (302) 366-1775
www.nursingworld.org/snas/de/

District of Columbia Nurses Association, Inc.
5100 Wisconsin Ave., N.W., Suite 306
Washington, D.C. 20016
(202) 244-2705
FAX (202) 362-8285

Florida Nurses Association
P.O. Box 536985
Orlando, Florida 32853-6985
(407) 896-3261
FAX (407) 896-9042
www.floridanurse.org

Georgia Nurses Association
1362 West Peachtree Street, N.W.
Atlanta, Georgia 30309
(404) 876-4624
FAX (404) 876-4621
www.nursingworld.org/snas/ga

Guam Nurses Association
P.O. Box CG
Hagatna, Guam 96932
Tel/Fax (671) 477-6877

Hawaii Nurses Association
677 Ala Moana Boulevard, Suite 301
Honolulu, Hawaii 96813
(808) 531-1628
FAX (808) 524-2760
www.hawaiinurses.org

Idaho Nurses Association
200 North 4th Street, Suite 20
Boise, Idaho 83702-6001
(208) 345-0500
FAX (208) 385-0166
www.nursingworld.org/snas/id

Illinois Nurses Association
105 West Adams St., suite 2101
Chicago, Illinois 60603
(312) 419-2900
FAX (312)419-292-
www.illinoisnurses.com

Indiana State Nurses Association
2915 North High School Road
Indianapolis, Indiana 46224
(317) 299-4575
FAX (317) 297-3525

Iowa Nurses Association
1501 42nd Street, Suite 471
West Des Moines, Iowa 50266
(515) 225-0495
FAX (515) 225-2201
www.iowanurses.org

Kansas State Nurses Association
1208 SW Tyler
Topeka, Kansas 66612-1735
(785) 233-8638
FAX (785) 233-5222
www.nursingworld.org/snas/ks

Kentucky Nurses Association
1400 South First Street
P.O. Box 2616
Louisville, Kentucky 40201
(502) 637-2546/2547
FAX (502) 637-8236
www.kentucky--nurses.org

Louisiana State Nurses Association
5700 Florida Blvd., Suite 720
Baton Rouge, Louisiana 70806
(225) 201-0993
(800) 457-6378
FAX (225) 201-0971
www.lsna.org

Maine State Nurses Association
P.O. Box 2240
295 Water Street
Augusta, Maine 04338-2240
(207) 622-1057
FAX (207) 623-4072
www.nursingworld.org/snas/me

Maryland Nurses Association
849 International Drive
Airport Square 21, Suite 255
Linthicum, Maryland 21090
(410) 859-3000
FAX (410) 859-3001
ww.nursingworld.org/snas/md

Massachusetts Nurses Association
340 Turnpike Street
Canton, Massachusetts 02021
(781) 821-4625
FAX (781) 821-4445
www.massnurses.org

Michigan Nurses Association
2310 Jolly Oak Road
Okemos, Michigan 48864-4599
(517) 349-5640
FAX (517) 349-5818
www.minurses.org

Minnesota Nurses Association
1625 Energy Park Drive
St. Paul, Minnesota 55108
(651) 646-4807
(800) 536-4662
FAX (651) 647-5301
www.mnnurses.org

Mississippi Nurses Association
31 Woodgreen Place
Madison, MS 39110
(601) 898-0670
FAX (601) 898-0190
www.msnurses.com

Missouri Nurses Association
1904 Bubba Lane, P.O. Box 105228
Jefferson City, Missouri 65110
1-888-662-MONA (toll-free)
(573) 636-4623
FAX (573) 636-9576
www.nursingworld.org/snas/mo/index.htm

Montana Nurses Association
104 Broadway, Suite G-2
Helena, Montana 59601
(406) 442-6710
FAX (406) 442-1841
www.nursingworld.org/snas/mt

Nebraska Nurses Association
715 South 14th Street
Lincoln, Nebraska 68508
(402) 475-3859
FAX(402) 475-3961
www.nursingworld.org/snas/ne/index.htm

Nevada Nurses Association
P.O. Box 530399
Henderson, Nevada 89053-0399
(702) 260-7886
FAX (702) 260-7052
www.nursingworld.org/snas/nv/index.htm

New Hampshire Nurses Association
48 West Street
Concord, New Hampshire 03301-3595
(603) 225-3783
FAX (603) 228-6672

New Jersey State Nurses Association
1479 Pennington Road
Trenton, New Jersey 08618-2661
(609) 883-5335, ext. 10
FAX (609) 883-5343
www.njsna.org

New Mexico Nurses Association
P.O. Box 80300
Albuquerque, New Mexico 87198
(505) 268-7744
FAX (505) 268-7711
www.nursingworld.org/snas/nm

New York State Nurses Association
11 Cornell Road
Latham, New York 12110
(518) 782-9400
FAX (518) 782-9530
www.nysna.org

North Carolina Nurses Association
103 Enterprise Street
Box 12025
Raleigh, North Carolina 27605
(919) 821-4250
FAX (919) 829-5807
www.nursingworld.org/snas/nc/index.htm

North Dakota Nurses Association
549 Airport Road
Bismarck, North Dakota 58504-6107
(701) 223-1385
FAX (701) 223-0575

Ohio Nurses Association
4000 East Main Street
Columbus, Ohio 43213-2983
1-800-430-0056
(614) 237-5414, ext. 1020
FAX (614) 237-6081
www.ohnurses.org

Oklahoma Nurses Association
6414 North Santa Fe, Suite A
Oklahoma City, Oklahoma 73116
(405) 840-3476
FAX (405) 840-3013
www.oknurses.com

Oregon Nurses Association
9600 SW Oak, Suite 550
Portland, Oregon 97223
(503) 293-0011
FAX (503) 293-0013
www.oregnrn.org

Pennsylvania State Nurses Association
P.O. Box 68525
Harrisburg, PA 17106-8525
(717) 657-1222
FAX (717) 657-3796
www.psna.org

Rhode Island State Nurses Association
550 S. Water Street, Unit 540B
Providence, RI 02903-4344
(401) 421-9703
FAX (401) 421-6793
www.risarn.org

South Carolina Nurses Association
1821 Gadsden Street
Columbia, South Carolina 29201
(803) 252-4781
FAX (803) 779-3870
www.nursingworld.org/snas/sc/index.htm

South Dakota Nurses Association
818 East 41st Street
Sioux Falls, South Dakota 57105
(605) 338-1401
FAX (605) 338-0516
www.nursingworld.org/snas/sd/index.htm

Tennessee Nurses Association
545 Mainstream Drive, Suite 405
Nashville, Tennessee 37228-1201
(615) 254-0350
FAX (615) 254-0303
www.tennurse.org

Texas Nurses Association
7600 Burnet Road, Suite 440
Austin, Texas 78757-1292
(512) 452-0645
FAX (512) 452-0648
www.texasnurses.org

Utah Nurses Association
3761 S. 700 East, #201
Salt Lake City, Utah 84106
(801) 293-8351
FAX (801) 293-8458
www.xmission.com:80/~una

Vermont State Nurses Association
100 Dorset Street, Suite 13
South Burlington, VT 05403
(802) 651-8888
FAX# (802) 651-8998
vtnurse@prodigy.net
www.nesna.org/html/vtnurses/vt.htm

Virgin Islands State Nurses Association
P.O. Box 583
Christiansted, St. Croix
U.S. Virgin Islands 00821-0583
(809) 773-1261

Virginia Nurses Association
7113 Three Chopt Road, Suite 204
Richmond, Virginia 23226
(804) 282-1808/2373
FAX (804) 282-4916
www.virginianurses.com

Washington State Nurses Association
575 Andover Park West, Suite 101
Seattle, Washington 98188-3321
(206) 575-7979
FAX (206) 575-1908
www.wsna.org

West Virginia Nurses Association
119 Summers Street
Charleston, West Virginia 25301
(304) 342-1169 or (800)400-1226
FAX (304) 342-6973
www.wvnurses.org

Wisconsin Nurses Association
6117 Monona Drive
Madison, Wisconsin 53716
(608) 221-0383
FAX (608) 221-2788
www.execpc.com/~wna/

Wyoming Nurses Association
Majestic Building, Room 305
1603 Capitol Avenue
Cheyenne, Wyoming 82001
(307) 635-3955
FAX (307) 635-2173
Office Hours: Tuesday/Friday 9:00am -1:00pm

Federal Nurses Association (FedNA)
www.nursingworld.org/FedNA

American Nurses Association
600 Maryland Avenue, SW
Suite 100W
Washington, DC 20024-2571
(202) 651-7000
(800) 274-4ANA
FAX (202) 651-7001
www.nursingworld.org

Constituent Assembly Executive Committee
American Nurses Association
600 Maryland Avenue, SW
Suite 100W
Washington, DC 20024-2571
(202) 651-7000
FAX (202) 651-7001

APPENDIX C

OSHA Contact Information: Area or Regional Offices

Region 1
Regional Office
JFK Federal Building, Room E340
Boston, Massachusetts 02203
(617) 565-9860
(617) 565-9827 FAX
Area Offices
Connecticut | Massachusetts | Maine |
New Hampshire | Rhode Island | Vermont

Region 2
Regional Office
201 Varick Street, Room 670
New York, New York 10014
(212) 337-2378
(212) 337-2371 FAX
Area Offices
New Jersey | New York | Puerto Rico | Virgin Islands

Region 3
Regional Office
Gateway Building, Suite 2100
3535 Market Street
Philadelphia, Pennsylvania 19104
(215) 596-1201
(215) 596-4872 FAX
Area Offices
District of Columbia | Delaware | Maryland |
Pennsylvania | Virginia | West Virginia

Region 4
Regional Office
61 Forsyth Street, SW
Atlanta, Georgia 30303
(404) 562-2300
(404) 562-2295 FAX
Area Offices
Alabama | Florida | Georgia | Kentucky | Mississippi
| North Carolina | South Carolina | Tennessee

Region 5
Regional Office
230 South Dearborn Street, Room 3244
Chicago, Illinois 60604
(312) 353-2220
(312) 353-7774 FAX
Area Offices
Illinois | Indiana | Michigan | Minnesota | Ohio
| Wisconsin

Region 6
Regional Office
525 Griffin Street, Room 602
Dallas, Texas
(214) 767-4731
(214) 767-4137 FAX
Area Offices
Arkansas | Louisiana | New Mexico | Oklahoma
| Texas

Region 7
Regional Office
City Center Square
1100 Main Street, Suite 800
Kansas City, Missouri 64105
(816) 426-5861
(816) 426-2750 FAX
Area Offices
Iowa | Kansas | Missouri | Nebraska

Region 8
Regional Office
1999 Broadway, Suite 1690
Denver, Colorado 80202-5716
(303) 844-1600
(303) 844-1616 FAX
Area Offices
Colorado | Montana | North Dakota | South Dakota
| Utah | Wyoming

Region 9
Regional Office
71 Stevenson Street, Room 420
San Francisco, California 94105
(415) 975-4310
(415) 744-4319 FAX
Area Offices
Arizona | California | Guam | Hawaii | Nevada

Region 10
Regional Office
1111 Third Avenue, Suite 715
Seattle, Washington 98101-3212
(206) 553-5930
(206) 553-6499 FAX
Area Offices
Alaska | Idaho | Oregon | Washington

APPENDIX D

OSHA-Approved State Occupational Safety and Health Plans

Alaska Department of Labor
1111 W. 8th Street, Room 306
Juneau, Alaska 99801
(907) 465-2720

Industrial Commission of Arizona
800 W. Washington
Phoenix, Arizona 85007
(602) 542-4653

California Department of Industrial Relations
45 Fremont Street
San Francisco, California 94105
(415) 703-5070

Connecticut Department of Labor
200 Folly Brook Boulevard
Wethersfield, Connecticut 06109
(860) 263-6000

Hawaii Department of Labor and Industrial Relations
830 Punchbowl Street
Honolulu, Hawaii 96813
(808) 586-8842

Indiana Department of Labor
State Office Building
402 West Washington Street, Room W195
Indianapolis, Indiana 46204
(317) 232-2655

Iowa Division of Labor Services
1000 E. Grand Avenue
Des Moines, Iowa 50319
(515) 284-4625

Kentucky Labor Cabinet
1047 U.S. Highway 127 South, Suite 2
Frankfort, Kentucky 40601
(502) 564-3075

Maryland Division of Labor and Industry
Department of Labor, Licensing and Regulation
1100 North Eutaw Street, Room 613
Baltimore, Maryland 21201-2206
(410) 631-3323

Michigan Department of Consumer and Industry Services
3423 North Martin Luther King Boulevard
P.O. Box 30649
Lansing, Michigan 48909
(517) 241-9313

Minnesota Department of Labor and Industry
443 Lafayette Road
St. Paul, Minnesota 55155
(651) 296-6107

Nevada Division of Industrial Relations
400 West King Street
Carson City, Nevada 97502
(775) 687-3032

New Mexico Environment Department
1190 St. Francis Drive
P.O. Box 26110
Santa Fe, New Mexico 87502
(505) 827-2855

New York Department of Labor
W. Averell Harriman State Office Building - 12, Room 500
Albany, New York 12240
(518) 457-5821

North Carolina Department of Labor
319 Chapanoke Road
Raleigh, North Carolina 27603
(919) 790-2801

Oregon Occupational Safety and Health Division
Department of Consumer and Business Services
350 Winter Street, NE, Room 430
Salem, Oregon 97310
(503) 378-3272

Puerto Rico Department of Labor and Human Resources
Prudencio Rivera Martinez Building
505 Munoz Rivera Avenue
Hato Rey, Puerto Rico 00918
(787) 754-5353

South Carolina Department of Labor, Licensing, and Regulation
Koger Office Park, Kingstree Building
110 Centerview Drive
PO Box 11329
Columbia, South Carolina 29210
(803) 896-4300

Tennessee Department of Labor
710 James Robertson Parkway
Nashville, Tennessee 37243-0659
Alphonso R. Bodie, Commissioner
(615) 741-2395

Labor Commission of Utah
160 East 300 South, 3rd Floor
PO Box 146650
Salt Lake City, Utah 84114-6650
R. Lee Ellertson, Commissioner
(801) 530-6851

Vermont Department of Labor and Industry
National Life Building - Drawer 20
120 State Street
Montpelier, Vermont 05620
Steve Janson, Commissioner
(802) 828-5098

Virginia Department of Labor and Industry Powers-Taylor Building
13 South 13th Street
Richmond, Virginia 23219
Theron Bell, Commissioner
(804) 786-3160

Virgin Islands Department of Labor
2131 Hospital Street
Box 890, Christiansted
St. Croix, Virgin Islands 00820-4666
Carmelo Rivera, Commissioner
(340) 773-1440

Washington Department of Labor and Industries
General Administration Building
PO Box 44001
Olympia, Washington 98504-4001
(360) 902-5269

Wyoming Department of Employment
Worker's Safety and Compensation Division
Herschler Building, 2nd Floor East
122 West 25th Street
Cheyenne, Wyoming 82002
(307) 235-3200

APPENDIX E

OSHA Consultation Services

ALABAMA
Safe State Program
University of Alabama
432 Martha Parham West
PO Box 870388
Tuscaloosa, Alabama 35487
(205) 348-3033
(205) 348-3049 FAX
bweems@ua.edu

ALASKA
ADOL/OSHA Division of Consultation
3301 Eagle Street
P.O. Box 107022
Anchorage, Alaska 99510
(907) 269-4957
(907) 269-4950 FAX
timothy_bundy@labor.state.ak.us

ARIZONA
Consultation and Training
Industrial Commission of Arizona
Division of Occupational Safety and Health
800 West Washington
Phoenix, Arizona 85007
(602) 542-5795
(602) 542-1614 FAX
henry@n245.osha.gov

ARKANSAS
OSHA Consultation
Arkansas Department of Labor
10421 West Markham
Little Rock, Arkansas 72205
(501) 682-4522
(501) 682-4532 FAX
clark@n237.osha.gov

CALIFORNIA
CAL/OSHA Consultation Service
Department of Industrial Relations
Room 1260
45 Freemont Street
San Francisco, California 94105
(415) 972-8515
(415) 972-8513 FAX
DCBare@hq.dir.ca.gov

COLORADO
Colorado State University
Occupational Safety and Health Section
115 Environmental Health Building
Fort Collins, Colorado 80523
(970) 491-6151
(970) 491-7778 FAX
rbuchan@lamar.colostate.edu

CONNECTICUT
Connecticut Department of Labor
Division of Occupational Safety and Health
38 Wolcott Hill Road
Wethersfield, Connecticut 06109
(203) 566-4550
(203) 566-6916 FAX
steve.wjeeter@ct-ce-wethrsfld.osha.gov

DELAWARE
Delaware Department of Labor
Division of Industrial Affairs
Occupational Safety and Health
4425 Market Street
Wilmington, Delaware 19802
(302) 761-8219
(302) 761-6601 FAX
ttrznadel@state.de.us

WASHINGTON, D.C.
DC Department of Employment Services
Office of Occupational Safety and Health
950 Upshur Street, N.W.
Washington, D.C. 20011
(202) 576-6339
(202) 576-7282 FAX
jcates@n217.osha.gov

FLORIDA
Florida Dept. of Labor and Employment Security
7(c)(1) Onsite Consultation Program Division
    of Safety
2002 St. Augustine Road, Building E,
Suite 45
Tallahassee, Florida 32399
(850) 922-8955
(850) 922-4538 FAX
brett_crecco@safety_fl.org

GEORGIA
7(c)(1) Onsite Consultation Program
Georgia Institute of Technology
O'Keefe Building, Room 22
Atlanta, Georgia 30332
(404) 894-2643
(404) 894-8275 FAX
paul.middendorf@gtri.gatech.edu

GUAM
OSHA Onsite Consultation
Dept. of Labor, Government of Guam
PO Box 9970
Tamuning, Guam 96931
(671) 475-0136
(671) 477-2988 FAX

HAWAII
Consultation and Training Branch
Dept of Labor and Industrial Relations
830 Punchbowl Street
Honolulu, Hawaii 96813
(808) 586-9100
(808) 586-9099 FAX

IDAHO
Boise State University, Dept. of Health Studies
1910 University Drive, ET-338A
Boise, Idaho 83725
(208) 385-3283
(208) 385-4411 FAX
lstokes@bsu.idbsu.edu

ILLINOIS
Illinois Onsite Consultation
Industrial Service Division
Department of Commerce and Community
Affairs
State of Illinois Center, Suite 3-400
100 West Randolph Street
Chicago, Illinois 60601
(312) 814-2337
(312) 814-7238 FAX
sfryzel@commerce.state.il.us

INDIANA
Bureau of Safety, Education and Training
Division of Labor, Room W195
402 West Washington
Indianapolis, Indiana 46204
(317) 232-2688
(317) 232-0748 FAX
jon.mack@nin-ce-indianpls.osha.gov

IOWA
7(c)(1) Consultation Program
Iowa Bureau of Labor
1000 East Grand Avenue
Des Moines, Iowa 50319
(515) 281-5352
(515) 281-4831 FAX

KANSAS
Kansas 7(c)(1) Consultation
Dept. of Human Resources
512 South West 6th Street
Topeka, Kansas 66603
(913) 296-7476
(913) 296-1775 FAX
rudy.leutzinger@ks-ce-topeka.gov

KENTUCKY
Division of Education and Training
Kentucky Labor Cabinet
1047 U.S. Highway 127 South
Frankfort, Kentucky 40601
(502) 564-6895
(502) 564-4769 FAX
arussell@mail.lab.state.ky.gov

LOUISIANA
7(c)(1) Consultation Program
Louisiana Department of Labor
OWC-OSHA Consultation
PO Box 94094
Baton Rouge, Louisiana 70804
(504) 342-9601
(504) 342-5158 FAX
oshacons@eatel.net

MAINE
Division of Industrial Safety
Maine Bureau of Labor
State House Station #82
Augusta, Maine 04333
(207) 624-6460
(207) 624-6449 FAX
david.e.wacker@state.me.us

MARYLAND
Division of Labor and Industry
312 Marshall Avenue, Room 600
Laurel, Maryland 20707
(410) 880-4970
(410) 880-6369 FAX

MASSACHUSETTS
The Commonwealth of Massachusetts
Dept. of Labor and Industries
1001 Watertown Street
West Newton, Massachusetts 02165
(617) 727-3982
(617) 727-4581 FAX
jlamalva@eol.state.ma.us

MICHIGAN (HEALTH)
Michigan Dept of Public Health
Division of Occupational Health
3423 North Martin Luther King Boulevard
Lansing, Michigan 48909
(517) 335-8250
(517) 335-8010 FAX
john.peck@cis.state.mi.us

MICHIGAN (SAFETY)
Michigan Dept of Consumer and Industry Services
7150 Harris Drive
Lansing, Michigan 48909
(517) 322-1809
(517) 322-1374 FAX
ayalew.kanno@cis.state.mi.us

MINNESOTA
Department of Labor and Industry
443 LaFayette Road
Saint Paul, Minnesota 55155
(612) 297-2393
(612) 297-1953 FAX
james.collins@state.mn.us

MISSISSIPPI
Mississippi State University
Center for Safety and Health
2906 North State Street, Suite 201
Jackson, Mississippi 39216
(601) 987-3981
(601) 987-3890 FAX
kelly.tucker@ms-c-jackson.osha.gov

MISSOURI
Division of Labor Standards Onsite Consultation Program
Department of Labor and Industrial Relations
3315 West Truman Boulevard
PO Box 449
Jefferson City, Missouri 65109
(573) 751-3403
(573) 751-3721 FAX
rsimmons@services.state.mo.us

MONTANA
Dept. of Labor and Industry Bureau of Safety
PO Box 1728
Helena, Montana 59624-1728
(406) 444-6418
(406) 444-4140 FAX
dfolsom@mt.gov

NEBRASKA
Division of Safety Labor and Safety Standards
Nebraska Department of Labor
State Office Building, Lower Level
301 Centennial Mall, South
Lincoln, Nebraska 68509-5024
(402) 471-4717
(402) 471-5039 FAX
amy@n214.osha.gov

NEVADA
Division of Preventive Safety
Department of Industrial Relations
Suite 106
2500 West Washington
Las Vegas, Nevada 89106
(702) 486-5016
(702) 486-5331 FAX
dalton.hooks@nv-ce-lasvegas.osha.gov

NEW HAMPSHIRE
New Hampshire Dept. of Health
Division of Public Health Services
6 Hazen Drive
Concord, New Hampshire 03301-6527
(603) 271-2024
(603) 271-2667 FAX
jake@nh7cl.mv.com

NEW JERSEY
New Jersey Department of Labor
Division of Public Safety and Occupational Safety and Health
225 E. State Street
8th Floor West
P.O. Box 953
Trenton, New Jersey 08625-0953
(609)292-3923
(609)292-4409 FAX
carol.farley@nj-c-trenton.osha.gov

NEW MEXICO
New Mexico Environment Department of Occupational Health and Safety Bureau
525 Camino de Los Marquez, Suite 3
PO Box 26110
Santa Fe, New Mexico 87502
(505) 827-4230
(505) 827-4422 FAX
deborah@n023.osha.gov

NEW YORK
Division of Safety and Health
State Office Campus
Building 12, Room 130
Albany, New York 12240
(518)457-1169
(518) 457-3454 FAX
james.rush@ny-ce-albany.osha.gov

NORTH CAROLINA
Bureau of Consultative Services
North Carolina Dept. of Labor
319 Chapanoke Road, Suite 105
Raleigh, North Carolina 27603-3432
(919) 662-4644
(919) 662-4671 FAX
wjoyner@mail.dol.state.nc.us

NORTH DAKOTA
Division of Environmental Engineering
1200 Missouri Avenue, Room 304
Bismarck, North Dakota 58504
(701) 328-5188
(701) 328-5200 FAX
cSNAil.domount@ranch.state.nd.us

OHIO
Bureau of Employment Services
145 S. Front Street
Columbus, Ohio 43216
(614) 644-2246
(614) 644-3133 FAX
owen@n222.osha.gov

OKLAHOMA
Oklahoma Department of Labor
OSHA Division
4001 North Lincoln Boulevard
Oklahoma City, Oklahoma 73105-5212
(405) 528-1500
(405) 528-5751 FAX
leslie@n238.osha.gov

OREGON
Department of Consumer and Business Services
Oregon Occupational Safety and Health Division
350 Winter Street NE, Room 430
Salem, Oregon 97310
(503) 378-3272
(800) 922-2689 Toll Free
(503) 378-5729 FAX
steve.g.beech@state.or.us *or* consult.web@state.or.us

PENNSYLVANIA
Indiana University of Pennsylvania
Safety Sciences Department
205 Uhler Hall
Indiana, Pennsylvania 15705-1087
(724) 357-2561
(724) 357-2385 FAX
dick@n196.osha.gov

PUERTO RICO
Occupational Safety and Health Office
Dept. of Labor and Human Resources, 21st Floor
505 Munoz Rivera Avenue
Hato Rey, Puerto Rico 00918
(787) 754-2171
(787) 767-6051 FAX
alopez@n114.osha.gov

RHODE ISLAND
Rhode Island Department of Health
Division of Occupational Health
3 Capital Hill
Providence, Rhode Island 02908
(401) 277-2438
(401) 277-6953 FAX
oshacon@ids.net

SOUTH CAROLINA
South Carolina Department of Labor
Licensing and Regulation
3600 Forest Drive
PO Box 11329
Columbia, South Carolina 29204
(803) 734-9614
(803) 734- 734-9741 FAX
scoshaovp@infoave.net

SOUTH DAKOTA
Engineering Extension
Onsite Technical Division
South Dakota State University
Box 510,
West Hall
907 Harvey Dunn Street
Brookings, South Dakota 57007
(605) 688-4101
(605) 688-6290 FAX
ceglian@ur.sdstate.edu

TENNESSEE
OSHA Consultative Services
Tennessee Department of Labor
710 James Robertson Parkway, 3rd Floor
Nashville, Tennessee 37243-0659
(615) 741-7036
(615) 532-2997 FAX
mike-maenza@tn-c-nashville.osha.gov

TEXAS
Workers' Health and Safety Division
Workers' Compensation Commission
Southfield Building
4000 South I H 35
Austin, Texas 78704
(512) 440-3854
(512) 440-3831 FAX
margaret.nugent@mail.capnet.state.tx.us

UTAH
Utah Industrial Commission
Consultation Services
160 East 300 South
Salt Lake City, Utah 84114-6650
(801) 530-6901
(801) 530-6992 FAX
iSNAin.nanderso@state.ut.us

VERMONT
Division of Occupational Safety and Health
Vermont Department of Labor and Industry
National Life Building, Drawer 20
Montpelier, Vermont 05602-3401
(802) 828-2765
(802) 828-2748 FAX
mcleod@labor.lab.state.vt.us

VIRGINIA
Virginia Department of Labor and Industry
Occupational Safety and Health Training and
  Consultation
13 South 13th Street
Richmond, Virginia 23219
(804) 786-6359
(804) 786-8418 FAX
njakubecdoli@sprintmail.com

VIRGIN ISLANDS
Division of Occupational Safety and Health
Virgin Islands Department of Labor
3021 Golden Rock
Christiansted
St. Croix, Virgin Island 00840
(809) 772-1315
(809) 772-4323 FAX

WASHINGTON
Washington Dept of Labor and Industries
Division of Industrial Safety and Health
PO Box 44643
Olympia, Washington 98504
(360) 902-5443
(360) 902-5459 FAX
jame235@lni.wa.gov

WEST VIRGINIA
West Virginia Department of Labor
Capitol Complex Building #3
1800 East Washington Street
Room 319
Charleston, West Virginia 25305
(304) 558-7890
(304) 558- 3797 FAX
jburgess@labor.state.wv.us

WISCONSIN (HEALTH)
Wisconsin Department of Health and Human
  Services
Section of Occupational Health
Room 112
1414 East Washington Avenue
Madison, Wisconsin 53703
(608) 266-8579
(608) 266-9711 FAX
moente@dhfs.state.wi.us

WISCONSIN (SAFETY)
Wisconsin Department of Industry
Labor and Human Relations
Bureau of Safety Inspections
401 Pilot Court, Suite C
Waukesha, Wisconsin 53188
(414) 521-5063
(414) 521-8614 FAX
jim.lutz@wi-c-waukesha.osha.gov

WYOMING
Wyoming Department of Employment
Workers' Safety and Compensation Division
Herschler Building, 2 East
122 West 25th Street
Cheyenne, Wyoming 82002
(307) 777-7786
(307) 777-3646 FAX
sfoste1@missc.state.wy.us

OTHER RELEVANT ADDRESSES

1908 Consultation Training Coordinator
OSHA Training Institute
1555 Times Drive
Des Plaines, Illinois 60018
(847) 297-4810

Laboratory Services
Wisconsin Occupational Health Lab
979 Johnathon Drive
Madison, Wisconsin 53713
(608) 263-8807
(608) 263-6551 FAX

New York Public Sector Consultation Program
New York State Department Of Labor
Building #12
State Building Campus
Albany, New York 12240
(518) 457-3518
(518) 457-5545 FAX

Director of Consultation Support Services
University of Alabama
College of Continuing Studies
425 Martha Parham West
Post Office Box 870388
Tuscaloosa, Alabama 35487-0388
(205) 348-4585
(205) 348-3049 FAX

APPENDIX F

OSHA Training Institute Education Centers

Region I - Keene State College
Robert Baker, Program Coordinator
Keene State College, Continuing Education Office
229 Main Street
Keene, New Hampshire 03435-2569
Phone: 800-449-6742
Phone: 603-358-2338
FAX: 603-358-2569
Web: www.keene.edu

Region II - Niagara County Community College
Raymond Z. Turpin, Coordinator
OSHA Training Institute Education Center
Niagara County Community College
Department of Corporate Training
136 Walnut Street
Lockport, New York 14094
Phone: 800-280-6742
Phone: 716-433-1856
FAX: 716-433-5155
E-mail: niagaraosha@wzrd.com
Web: www.sunyniagara.cc.ny.us

Region III - The National Resource Center for OSHA Training
James Strother, Director
The National Resource Center for OSHA Training
815 16th Street, N.W., Room #603
Washington, D.C. 20006
Phone: 800-367-6724
FAX: 202-628-0724
E-mail: jtstrother@radix.net
Web: www.wvu.edu/~exten/she/osha.htm

Region IV - Georgia Tech Research Institute
Daniel J. Ortiz, Manager
Safety, Health, and Ergonomics Branch
Electro-Optics, Environment, and Materials Lab
Georgia Tech Research Institute
151 Sixth Street
Atlanta, Georgia 30332-0800
Phone: 800-653-3629
Phone: 404-894-8276
FAX: 404-894-8275
Web: www.gatech.edu

Region V - Great Lakes Regional OSHA
Training Consortium
Jeanne F. Ayers, Director
Program in Continuing Education
Midwest Center for Occupational Health and Safety
640 Jackson Street
St. Paul, Minnesota 55101
Phone: 800-493-2060
Phone: 612-221-3980
FAX: 612-292-4773
Web: www.healthpartners.com/mcohs/mcohs.html

Region V - Eastern Michigan UAW OSHA
Education Center
Beth Stoner, Institute Administrator
Center for Organizational Risk Reduction
Eastern Michigan University
2000 Huron River Drive, Suite 101
Ypsilanti, Michigan 48197
Phone: 800-932-8689
Phone: 313-487-6988
FAX: 313-481-0509
E-mail: Beth.Stoner@emich.edu
Web: www.emich.edu/public/osha

Region V - The National Safety Education Center
Deborah Brue, Director
Office of External Programming
College of Engineering and Engineering Technology
Engineering Building, Room 318
Northern Illinois University
DeKalb, Illinois 60115
Phone: 800-656-5317
Phone: 815-753-6902
FAX: 815-753-4203
E-mail: brue@ceet.niu.edu
Web: www.ceet.niu.edu/extprg/index.html

Region VI - Southwest Education Center
Teresea Madden-Thompson, Associate Director
OSHA Training Institute
Southwest Education Center
Texas Engineering Extension Service
The Texas A and M University System
15515 IH-20 at Lumley
Mesquite, Texas 75181
Phone: 800-723-3811
FAX: 972-222-6704
E-mail: adthomps@teexnet.tamu.edu

Region VII - Maple Woods Community College
Dick Holzrichter, Industrial/Technical Training
  Supervisor
Maple Woods Community College
7703 N.W. Barry Road
Kansas, City, Missouri 64153
Phone: 800-841-7158
Phone: 816-741-0711
FAX: 816-587-3747

Region VIII - Rocky Mountain Education Center
Richard Hawkins, Director
OSHA Training Institute
Rocky Mountain Education Center
OSHA - Campus Box 41
Red Rocks Community College
13300 West Sixth Avenue
Lakewood, Colorado 80401-5398
Phone: 800-933-8394
Phone: 303-914-6420
FAX: 303-980-8339

Region IX - Pacific Coast Training Center
Michael Gall, Executive Director
OSHA Training Institute Education Center
University of California, San Diego
15373 Innovation Drive, Suite 105
San Diego, California 92128-3424
Phone: 800-358-9206
Phone: 619-451-7695
FAX: 619-485-7390
E-mail: mgall@ucsd.edu

Region X - University of Washington
Jan Schwert, Manager
Continuing Education Program
Department of Environmental Health
University of Washington
4225 Roosevelt Way NE, Suite 100
Seattle, Washington 98105-6099
Phone: 800-326-7568
Phone: 206-543-8068
FAX: 206-685-3872
E-mail: jschwert@u.washington.edu
Web Site - www.sphcm.washington.edu/
  DEHWeb/ce_osha.html

OSHA Training Education Centers Consortium Contacts

**Region III - The National Resource Center for
  OSHA Training**
Paul Becker, Program Leader
University of West Virginia
Safety and Health Extension
130 Tower Lane, P.O. Box 6615
Morgantown, West Virginia 26506-6615
Phone: 800-626-4748
Phone: 304-293-3096
FAX: 304-293-5905
E-mail: PBecker@WVNVMS.WVNET.edu

Janice Wheeler, OSHA Training Coordinator
Occupational Health Foundation
815 16th Street, N.W., Room 312
Washington, D.C. 20006
Phone: 202-842-7840
FAX: 202-842-7806

**Region V - Great Lakes OSHA Training Con-
sortium**
Regina Hoffman, Director
Continuing Education
Minnesota Safety Council
474 Concordia Avenue
St. Paul, Minnesota 55103
Phone: 800-444-9150
Phone: 612-291-9150
FAX: 612-291-7584

Judy L. Jarrell, Ed.D., MA
Director, ERC Continuing Education
University of Cincinnati
Department of Environmental Health
P.O. Box 670056
Cincinnati, Ohio 45267-0056
Phone: 800-207-9399
Phone: 513-558-1730
FAX: 513-558-1756
E-mail: judy.jarrell@uc.edu

**Region V - The National Safety Education
  Center**
Thomas A. Broderick, Executive Director
Construction Safety Council
4415 West Harrison Street, Suite 403
Hillside, Illinois 60162
Phone: 800-552-7744
Phone: 708-449-0200
FAX: 708-449-0369

Don Ostrander, CSP Manager
Safety and Health Management Services
National Safety Council
1121 Spring Lake Drive
Itasca, Illinois 60143-3201
Phone: 800-621-7615
Phone: 708-775-2341
FAX: 708-775-2185

APPENDIX G

OSHA Publications

Employee Workplace Rights (OSHA 3021)

Acute Care Facilities (OSHA 3128)

Bloodborne Pathogens and Long-Term Care Workers (OSHA 3131)

Chemical Hazard Communication (OSHA 3084)

Ergonomic Guidelines For Meatpacking Plants (OSHA 3123)

Guidelines For Preventing Workplace Violence For Health Care And Social Service Workers (OSHA 3148)

Framework for a Comprehensive Health and Safety Program in the Hospital Environment (1993)

Framework for a Comprehensive Health and Safety Program in Nursing Homes (1996)

OSHA Fact Sheets

Access To Employee Exposure and Medical Records

Back Injuries: Nation's Number One Workplace Safety Pproblem

Bloodborne Pathogens Final Standard

Enforcement Policy on Tuberculosis

General OSHA Recordkeeping Requirements

Hazard Communication Standard

Improving Workplace Protection for New Workers Inspecting for Job Safety and Health Hazards Job Safety and Health

OSHA Emergency Hot-line OSHA Facts: Common Sense at Work.

Protecting Community Workers Against Violence

Responding to Workplace Emergencies

Safety with Video Display Terminals

Single, free copies of OSHA publications can be obtained from the following sources:
   U.S. Department of Labor
   OSHA Publications
   PO Box 37535
   Washington, DC 20013-7535
   (202) 219-4667
   fax (202) 219-9266

OSHA Web site at www.osha.gov
(At the OSHA home page, go to Newsroom and click on <pubs>.)

APPENDIX H

NIOSH Publications

National Institute for Occupational Safety and Health
Centers for Disease Control and Prevention
1600 Clifton Road
Atlanta, GA 30333
1-800-35NIOSH or 1-800-356-4674

NIOSH has published numerous documents that are relevant to the health and safety of health care workers, ranging from technical reports to educational documents. To request any of these publications, you can:

■ Call NIOSH at 1-800-356-4674

■ Visit their web site at http://www.cdc.gov/niosh/pubs.html

■ Send your request via e-mail to pubstaft@cdc.gov or via fax to (513) 533-8573

■ Mail your order to:
  NIOSH Publications
  4676 Columbia Parkway, Mail Stop C-13
  Cincinnati, OH 45226-1998

Title	Publication #
NIOSH Alert: Preventing Needlestick Injuries in Health Care Settings	2000-108
Respiratory Protection Program in Health Care Facilities: Administrator's Guide	99-143
Control of Nitrous Oxide During Cryosurgery (Hazard Control 29)	99-105
The Effects of Workplace Hazards on Female Reproductive Health	99-104
Stress at Work	99-101
Joint FDA/NIOSH/OSHA Advisory on Glass Capillary Tubes: Joint Safety Advisory About Potential Risks	2/22/99
Latex Allergy: A Prevention Guide	98-113
NIOSH Alert: Preventing Allergic Reactions to Natural Rubber Latex in the Workplace	97-135
Selecting, Evaluating, and Using Sharps Disposal Containers	97-111
The Effects of Workplace Hazards on Male Reproductive Health	96-132
Control of Smoke From Laser/Electric Surgical Procedures (Hazard Control 11)	96-128
Protect Yourself Against Tuberculosis: A Respiratory Protection Guide for Health Care Workers	96-102

APPENDIX I

NIOSH Education and Research Center (ERCs)

Alabama Education and Research Center
University of Alabama at Birmingham
School of Public Health
Birmingham, AL 35294-0008
(205) 934-8488

**California Education and Research Center:
Northern**
University of California at Berkeley
School of Public Health
140 Warren
Berkeley, CA 94720-7360
(510) 642-0761

**California Education and Research Center:
Southern**
University of Southern California
School of Medicine
Department of Preventive Medicine
1540 Alcazar Street
Suite 236
Los Angeles, CA 90033
(213) 342-1096

Cincinnati Education and Research Center
University of Cincinnati
Department of Environmental Health
P.O. Box 670056
Cincinnati, Ohio 45267-0056
(513) 558-1749

Harvard Education and Research Center
Harvard School of Public Health
Department of Environmental Health
665 Huntington Avenue
Boston, MA 02115
(617) 432-3323

Illinois Education and Research Center
University of Illinois at Chicago
School of Public Health
2121 West Taylor Street M/C 922
Chicago, IL 60612-7260
(312) 996-7887

Johns Hopkins Education and Research Center
Johns Hopkins University
School of Hygiene and Public Health
615 North Wolfe Street
Baltimore, MD 21205
(410) 955-4082

Michigan Education and Research Center
University of Michigan
College of Engineering
Dept. of Industrial and Operations
Engineering Building
1205 Beal Avenue
Ann Arbor, MI 48109
(313) 763-0563

Minnesota Education and Research Center
University of Minnesota
School of Public Health
Minneapolis, MN 55455
(612) 626-0900

**New York/New Jersey Education and Research
Center**
Department of Community Medicine
Mt. Sinai School of Medicine
P.O. Box 1057
One Gustave L. Levy Pl.
New York, NY 10029-6574
(212) 241-4804

North Carolina Education and Research Center
University of North Carolina
School of Public Health
Rosenau Hall, CB# 7400
Chapel Hill, NC 27599-7400
(919) 966-3473

South Florida Education and Research Center
University of South Florida
College of Public Health
13201 Bruce B. Downs Blvd., MDC Box 56
Tampa, FL 33612-3805
(813) 974-6626

Texas Education and Research Center
The University of Texas Health Science
Center at Houston
School of Public Health
P.O. Box 20186
Houston, TX 77225-0186
(713) 500-9459

Utah Education and Research Center
University of Utah
Rocky Mountain Center for Occupational and
    Environmental Health, Bldg. 512
Salt Lake City, UT 84112
(801) 581-8719

Washington Education and Research Center
University of Washington
Department of Environmental Health
P.O. Box 357234
Seattle, WA 98195-7234
(206) 543-6991

APPENDIX J

COSH and Other Occupational Health and Safety Groups

Listed below are Committees for Occupational Safety and Health groups and related groups that provide educational and technical health and safety services. Also listed in this appendix are the national offices of key professional occupational health and safety associations.

ALASKA
Alaska Health Project
218 East 4th Ave.
Anchorage, AK 99501
(907) 276-2864
Fax: 907-279-3089

CALIFORNIA
Worksafe/Francis Schreiberg
C/o San Francisco Labor Council
1188 Franklin St, Suite 203
San Francisco, CA 94109
(415) 433-5077 (messages only)
Fax: 510-835-4913
Fcs@kmes.com

LACOSH (Los Angeles)
5855 Venice Blvd.
Los Angeles, CA 90019
(213) 931-9000
Fax: 213-931-2255

SA-COSH (Sacramento)
c/o Fire Fighters Local 522
3101 Stockton Blvd
Sacramento, CA 95820
(916) 442-4390
Fax: 916-446-3057

SCCOSH (Santa Clara)
760 N. 1st St., 2nd floor
San Jose, CA 95112
(408) 998-4050
Fax: 408-998-4051
sccosh@igc.org

CONNECTICUT
ConnectiCOSH
77 Huyshope Ave., 2nd floor
Hartford, CT 06106
(860) 549-1877
Fax: 860-251-6049
connecticosh@snet.net

ILLINOIS
CACOSH (Chicago Area)
C/o Mike Ross
UIC School of Public Health
Great Lakes Center, M/C-922
2121 West Taylor St.
Chicago, IL 60612-7260
(312) 996-2747
Fax: 312-413-7369
cacosh@hotmail.com

MAINE
Maine Labor Group on Health
Box V
Augusta, ME 04330
(207) 622-7823
Fax: (207) 622-3483 or 207-623-4916

MARYLAND
Alice Hamilton Occupational Health Center
1310 Apple Avenue
Silver Spring, MD 20910-3354
301-565-4590
Fax: 301-565-4596/97
bc74@telnet.umd.edu

MASSACHUSETTS
MassCOSH
555 Amory St.
Boston, MA 02130
(617) 524-6686
Fax: 617-524-3508
masscosh@shore.net

Western MassCOSH
458 Bridge Street
Springfield, MA 01103
413-731-0760
Fax: 413-731-6688
masscosh@external.umass.edu

MICHIGAN
SEMCOSH (Southeast Michigan)
1550 Howard St.
Detroit, MI 48216
(313) 961-3345
Fax: (313) 961-3588
semcosh@mich.com

MINNESOTA
MnCOSH
C/o Lyle Krych
5013 Girard Avenue North
Minneapolis, MN 55430
(612) 572-6997
Fax: (612) 572-9826

NEW HAMPSHIRE
NHCOSH
110 Sheep Davis Road
Pembroke, NH 03275
(603) 226-0516
Fax: (603) 225-1956

NEW YORK
ALCOSH (Alleghany)
20 West 3rd Street, Suite 21
Jamestown, NY 14701
(716) 488-0720
Fax: (716) 487-0968

CNYCOSH (Central NY)
615 W. Genessee St.
Syracuse, NY 13204
(315) 471-6187
Fax: (315) 471-6193

ENYCOSH (Eastern NY)
C/o Larry Rafferty
121 Erie Blvd
Schenectady, NY 12305
(518) 372-4308
Fax: (518) 393-3040

NYCOSH (NYC)
275 Seventh Ave, 8th Floor
NY, NY 10001
(212) 627-3900
Fax: (212) 627-9812
nycosh@compuserve.com

ROCOSH (Rochester)
46 Prince St.
Rochester, NY 14607
(716) 244-0420
Fax: (716) 244-0956
spula@dbi.cc.rochester.edu or
billbenet@aol.com

WNYCOSH (Western NY)
2495 Main Street, Suite 438
Buffalo, NY 14214
(716) 833-5416
Fax: (716) 833-7507
jbieger@pce.net

NORTH CAROLINA
NCOSH
PO Box 2514
Durham, NC 27715
(919) 286-9249
Fax: (919) 286-4857
ncosh@igc.apc.org

OREGON
ICWU-Portland
c/o Dick Edgington
7440 SW 87 Street
Portland, OR 97223
(503) 244-8429 – No Fax

PENNSYLVANIA
PHILAPOSH (Philadelphia)
3001 Walnut St., 5th Floor
Philadelphia, PA 19104
(215) 386-7000
Fax: (215) 386-3529
philaposh@aol.com

RHODE ISLAND
RICOSH
741 Westminster St.
Providence, RI 02903
(401) 751-2015
Fax: (401) 751-7520

TEXAS
TexCOSH
C/o Karyl Dunson
5735 Regina
Beaumont, TX 77706
(409) 898-1427 –No Fax

WISCONSIN
WisCOSH
734 N. 26th St.
Milwaukee, WI 53230
(414) 933-2338
Fax: (414) 342-1998
wiscoshm@it is.com

CANADA (Ontario)
WOSH (Windsor)
547 Victoria Avenue
Windsor, Ontario N9A 4N1
(519) 973-4800
Fax: (519) 973-1906
jbrophy@mnsi.net

COSH Related Groups

CALIFORNIA
Labor Occupational Health Program
2223 Fulton St, 4th Floor
Berkeley, CA 94720-5120
(510) 642-5507
Fax: (510) 643-5698
lstock@uclink4.berkeley.edu

UCLA-LOSH Program
School of Public Policy and Social Research
Inst. Of Industrial Relations
6350 B Public Policy Bldg.
Box 951478
Los Angeles, CA 90095-1478
(310) 794-5964
Fax: (310) 794-6410

DISTRICT OF COLUMBIA
Workers Institute for Occupational Safety and
   Health
1126 16th St., NW, Rm. 403
Washington, DC 20036
(202) 887-1980
Fax: (202) 887-0910

LOUISIANA
Labor Studies Program/LA Watch
Institute of Human Relations
Loyola University, Box 12
New Orleans, LA 70118
(504) 861-5830
Fax: (504) 861-5833

MASSACHUSETTS
Massachusetts Coalition on New Office
   Technology (CNOT)
650 Beacon St., 5th Floor
Boston, MA 02215
(617) 247-6827
Fax: (617) 262-6414

MICHIGAN
Michigan Right-to-Act Campaign
Ecology Center of Ann Arbor
417 Detroit St.
Ann Arbor, MI 48104
(313) 633-2404
Fax: (313) 633-2414
hnixon6081@aol.com
local223@aol.com

NEW JERSEY
New Jersey Work Environment Council
452 East Third Street
Moorestown, NJ 08057
(606) 866-9405
Fax: (606) 866-9708

NEW YORK
Midstate Central Labor Coalition
109 West State St.
Ithaca, NY 14850
(607) 277-5670 –No Fax
chf6@cornell.edu

OHIO
Greater Cincinnati Occupational Health Center
311 Howell Ave., Lower Level
Cincinnati, OH 45220
(513) 569-0561

WEST VIRGINIA
Institute of Labor Studies
710 Knapp Hall
West Virginia University
Morgantown, WV 26506
(304) 293-3323
Fax: (304) 293-7163

CANADA
Windsor Occupational Health Information
   Service
547 Victoria Ave.
Windsor, Ontario N9A 4N1
(519) 254-5157
Fax: (519) 254-4192
wohis@mnsi.net

ENGLAND
London Hazards Centre Interchange Studios
Dalby Street
London, England NW5 3NQ
Phone: 0171 267-3387
Fax: 0171 267-3397
lonhaz@mcr1.poptel.org.uk

WHIN – Workers Health International
   Newsletter and HAZARDS Magazine
PO Box 199
Sheffield, England S1 4YL
Phone: +44 114 276-5695
Fax: +44 114 276-7257
whin-hazards@mcr1.poptel.org.uk

Professional Occupational Health and Safety Associations

These national associations have state and local chapters that can be of assistance. Contact the national offices for a referral.

AAOHN, Inc.
American Association of Occupational Health Nurses
Suite 100, 2920 Brandywine Road,
Atlanta, GA 30341
(770) 455-7757 Fax (770) 455-7271
www.aaohn.org

AIHA
American Industrial Hygiene Association
2700 Prosperity Avenue
Suite 250
Fairfax, VA 22031
Phone: (703) 849-8888 Fax: (703) 207-3561
E-Mail: infonet@aiha.org InfoFax Service:
(703) 641-INFO
www.aiha.org

AOHP
Association of Occupational Health Professionals in Healthcare
11250 Roger Bacon Drive
Suite 8
Reston, Virginia 20190-5202
(800) 362-4347 or (703) 43704377
Fax: (703) 435-4390
www.aohp.org/aohp/

AOEC
Association of Occupational and Environmental Clinics
1030 15th St. NW #410
Washington, D.C. 20005
(202) 682-1807

APHA
American Public Health Association, Inc.
1015 15th St. NW
Washington, DC 2005-2605
(202) 789-5600
Fax: (202) 789-7661
www.apha.org

APIC
Association for Professionals in Infection Control and Epidemiology, Inc.
P.O. Box 79502
Baltimore, MD 21279-0502.
(202) 296-2742
Fax (202) 296-5645
www.apic.org

ASSE
American Society of Safety Engineers
1800 E. Oakton St.,
Des Plaines, IL 60018
Phone: (847) 699-2929
www.asse.org

IOSH
The Institution of Occupational Safety and Health
The Grange
Highfield Drive
Wigston, Leicestershire, LE18 1NN
United Kingdom
Tel: +44 (0)116 257 3100,
Fax: +44 (0)116 257 3101
www.iosh.co.uk

Other Resources

Joint Commission on Accreditation of Healthcare Organizations (JCAHO) www.jcaho.org

To order these publications:

- *Environment of Care: Essentials for Health Care* (ECE01SJ)
- *Environment of Care: Handbook* (EC100SJ)
- *Managing Indoor Air Quality in Healthcare Organizations* (EC505SJ)

either go to http://www.jcaho.org/lwapps/online/frntgt_frm.html or call 630-792-5800.

APPENDIX K

OSHA Form No. 101

Occupational Safety and Health Administration
Supplementary Record of
Occupational Injuries and Illnesses

U.S. Department of Labor

This form is required by Public Law 91-596 and must be kept in the establishment for 5 years.
Failure to maintain can result in the issuance of citations and assessment of penalties.

Case or File No.

Form Approved
O.M.B. No. 1218-0176

See OMB Disclosure
Statement on reverse.

Employer

1. Name

2. Mail address (No. and street, city or town, State, and zip code)

3. Location, if different from mail address

Injured or Ill Employee

4. Name (First, middle, and last)

Social Security No.

5. Home address (No. and street, city or town, State, and zip code)

6. Age

7. Sex (Check one) Male ☐ Female ☐

8. Occupation (Enter regular job title, not the specific activity he was performing at the time of injury.)

9. Department (Enter name of department or division in which the injured person is regularly employed, even though he may have been temporarily working in another department at the time of injury.)

The Accident or Exposure to Occupational Illness

If accident or exposure occurred on employer's premises, give address of plant or establishment in which it occurred. Do not indicated department or division within the plant or establishment. If accident occurred outside employer's premises at an identifiable address, give that address. If it occurred on a public highway or at any other place which cannot be identified by number and street, please provide place references locating the place of injury as accurately as possible.

10. Place of accident or exposure (No. and street, city or town, State, and zip code)

11. Was place of accident or exposure on employer's premises? Yes ☐ No ☐

12. What was the employee doing when injured? (Be specific. If he was using tools or equipment or handling material, name them and tell what he was doing with them.)

13. How did the accident occur? (Describe fully the events which resulted in the injury or occupational illness. Tell what happened and how it happened. Name any objects or substances involved and tell how they were involved. Give full details on all factors which led or contributed to the accident. Use separate sheet for additional space.)

Occupational Injury or Occupational Illness

14. Describe the injury or illness in detail and indicate the part of body affected. (E.g., amputation of right index finger at second joint; fracture of ribs; lead poisoning; dermatitis of left hand, etc.)

15. Name the object or substance which directly injured the employee. (For example, the machine or thing he struck against or which struck him; the vapor or poison he inhaled or swallowed; the chemical or radiation which irriatated his skin; or in cases of strains, hernias, etc., the thing he was lifting, pulling, etc.)

16. Date of injury or initial diagnosis of occupational illness

17. Did employee die? (Check one) Yes ☐ No ☐

Other

18. Name and address of physician

19. If hospitalized, name and address of hospital

Date of report

Prepared by

Official position

OSHA No. 101 (Feb. 1981)

(See Next Page/Reverse)

APPENDIX L

Instructions for OSHA 200 Log

OMB DISCLOSURE STATEMENT

Instructions for OSHA No. 200

I. Log and Summary of Occupational Injuries and Illnesses

Each employer who is subject to the recordkeeping requirements of the Occupational Safety and Health Act of 1970 must maintain for each establishment, a log of all recordable occupational injuries and illnesses. This form (OSHA No. 200) may be used for that purpose. A substitute for the OSHA No. 200 is acceptable if it is as detailed, easily readable, and understandable as the OSHA No. 200.

Enter each recordable case on the log within six (6) workdays after learning of its occurrence. Although other records must be maintained at the establishment to which they refer, it is possible to prepare and maintain the log at another location, using data processing equipment if desired. If the log is prepared elsewhere, a copy updated to within 45 calendar days must be present at all times in the establishment.

Logs must be maintained and retained for five (5) years following the end of the calendar year to which they relate. Logs must be available (normally at the establishment) for inspection and copying by representatives of the Department of Labor, or the Department of Health and Human Services, or States accorded jurisdiction under the Act. Access to the log is also provided to employees, former employees and their representatives.

II. Changes in Extent of or Outcome of Injury or Illness

If, during the 5-year period the log must be retained, there is a change in an extent and outcome of an injury or illness which affects entries in columns 1, 2, 6, 8, 9, or 13, the first entry should be lined out and a new entry made. For example, if an injured employee at first required only medical treatment but later lost workdays away from work, the check in column 6 should be lined out and checks entered in columns 2 and 3 and the number of lost workdays entered in column 4.

In another example, if an employee with an occupational illness lost wordays, returned to work, and then died of the illness, any entries in columns 9 through 12 would be lined out and the date of death entered in column 8.

The entire entry for an injury or illness should be lined out if later found to be nonrecordable. For example, an injury which is later determined not to be work related, or which was initially thought to involve medical treatement but later was determined to have involved only first aid.

III. Posting Requirements

A copy of the totals and information following the total line of the last page for the year, must be posted at each establishment in the place or places where notices to employees are customarily posted. This copy must be posted no later than February 1 and must remain in place until March 1. Even though there were no injuries or illnessed during the year, zeros must be entered on the totals line, and the form posted.

The person responsible for the annual summary totals shall certify that the totals are true and complete by signing at the bottom of the form.

IV. Instructions for Completing Log and Summary of Occupational injuries and illnesses

Column A - CASE OR FILE NUMBER. Self Expanatory

Column B - DATE OF INJURY OR ONSET OF ILLNESS

For occupational injuries, enter the date of the work accident which resulted in the injury. For occupational illnesses, enter the date of initial diagnosis of illness, or, if absence from work occurred before diagnosis, enter the first day of the absence attributable to the illness which was later diagnosed or recognized.

Columns C through F - Self Explanatory

Columns 1 and 8 - INJURY OR ILLNESS-RELATED DEATHS - Self Explanatory

Columns 2 and 9 - INJURIES OR ILLNESSES WITH LOST WORKDAYS - Self Explanatory

Any injury which involves days away from work, or days of restricted work activitiy, or both, must be recorded since it always involves one or more of the criteria for recordability.

Columns 3 and 10 - INJURIES OR ILLNESSES INVOLVING DAYS AWAY FROM WORK - Self Explanatory

Columns 4 and 11 - LOST WORKDAYS -- DAYS AWAY FROM WORK.
Enter the number of workdays (consecutive or not) on which the employee would have worked but could not because of occupational injury or illness. The number of lost workdays should not include the day of injury or onset of illness or any days on which the employee would not have worked even though able to work. NOTE: For employees not having a regularly scheduled shift, such as certain truck drivers, construction workers, farm labor, casual labor, part-time employees, etc., it may be necessary to estimate the number of lost workdays. Estimates of lost workdays shall be based on prior work history of the employee AND days worked by employees, not ill or injured, working in the department and/or occupation of the ill or injured employee.

Columns 5 and 12 - LOST WORKDAYS -- DAYS OF RESTRICTED WORK ACTIVITY.
Enter the number of workdays (consecutive or not) on which because of injury or illness:
(1) the employee was assigned to another job on a temporary basis, or
(2) the employee worked at a permanent job less than full time, or
(3) the employee worked at a permanently assigned job but could not perform all duties normally connected with it.

The number of lost workdays should not include the day of injury or onset of illness or any days on which the employee would not have worked even though able to work.

Columns 6 and 13 - INJURIES OR ILLNESSES WITHOUT LOST WORKDAYS - Self Explanatory

Columns 7a through 7g - TYPE OF ILLNESS. Enter a check in only *one* column for each illness.
TERMINATION OR PERMANENT TRANSFER - Place an asterisk to the right of the entry in columns 7a through 7g (type of illness) which represented a termination of employment or permanent transfer.

V. Totals
Add number of entries in columns 1 and 8.
Add number of checks in columns 2, 3, 6, 7, 9, 10 and 13.
Add number of days in columns 4, 5, 11 and 12.
Yearly totals for each column (1-13) are required for posting. Running or page totals may be generated at the discretion of the employer.

In an employee's loss of workdays is continuing at the time the totals are summarized, estimate the number of future workdays the employee will lose and add that estimate to the workdays already lost and include this figure in the annual totals. No further entries are to be made with respect to such cases in the next year's log.

VI. Definitions
OCCUPATIONAL INJURY is any injury such as a cut, fracture, sprain, amputation, etc. which results from a work accident or from an exposure involving a single incident in the work environment. NOTE: Conditions resulting from animal bites, such as insect or snake bites or from one-time exposure to chemicals, are considered to be injuries.

OCCUPATIONAL ILLNESS of an amployee is any abnormal condition or disorder, other than one resulting from an occupational injury, caused by exposure to environmental factors associated with employment. It includes acute and chronic illnesses or diseases which may be caused by inhalation, absorption, ingestion, or direct contact.

The following listing gives the categories of occupational illnesses and disorders that will be utilized for the purpose of classifying recordable illnesses. For porposes of information, examples of each category are given. These are typical examples, however, and are not to be considered the complete listing of the types of illnesses and disorders that are to be counted under each category.

7a. Occupational Skin Diseases or Disorders. Examples: Contact dermatitis, eczema, or rash caused by primary irritants and sensitizers or poisonous plants; oil acne; chrome ulcers; chemical burns or inflamation, etc.

7b. Dust Diseases of the Lungs (Pneumaconioses). Examples: Silicosis, asbestosis and other asbestos-related diseases, coal worker's pneumaconioses, byssinosis, siderosis, and other pneumaconioses.

7c. Respiratory Conditions Due to Toxic Agents. Examples: Pneumonitis, pharyngitis, rhinitis or acute congestion due to chemicals, dusts, gases, or fumes; farmer's lung; etc.

7d. Poisoning (Systemic Effects of Toxic Materials). Examples: Poisoning by lead, mercury, cadmium, arsenic, or other metals; poisoning by carbon monoxide, hydrogen sulfide, or other gases; poisoning by benzol, carbon tetrachloride, or other organic solvents; poisoning by insecticide sprays such as parathion, lead arsenate; poisoning by other chemicals such as formaldehyde, plastics, and resins; etc.

7e. Disorders Due to Physical Agents (Other than Toxic Materials). Examples: Heatstroke, sunstroke, heat exhaustion, and other effects of environmental heat, freezing, frostbite, and effects of exposure to low temperatures; caisson disease; effects of ionizing radiation (isotopes, X-rays, radium); effects of nonionizing radiation (welding flash, ultraviolet rays, microwaves, sunburn); etc.

7f. Disorders Associated with Repeated Trauma. Examples: Noise-induced hearing loss; synovitis, tenosynovitis, and bursitis. Raynaud's phenomena; and other conditions due to repeated motion, vibration, or pressure.

7g. All Other Occupational Illnesses. Examples: Anthrax, brucellosis, infectious hepatitis, malignant and benign tumors, food poisoning, histoplasmosis, coccidioidomycosis, etc.

MEDICAL TREATMENT includes treatment (other than first aid) administered by a physician or by registered professional personnel under the standing orders of a physician. Medical treatment does NOT include first aid treatment (one-time treatment and subsequent observation of minor scratches, cuts, burns, splinters, and so forth, which do not ordinarily require medical care) even though provided by a physician or registered professional personnel.

ESTABLISHMENT: A single physical location where business is conducted or where services or industrial operations are performed (for example: a factory, mill, store, hotel, resturant, movie theater, farm, ranch, bank, sales office, warehouse, or central administrative office). Where distinctly separate activities are performed at a single physicial location, such as construction activities operated from the same physical locations as a lumber yard, each activity shall be treated as a separate establishment.

For firms engaged in activities which may be physically dispersed, such as agriculture; construction; transportation; communications and electric, gas, and sanitary services, records may be maintained at a place to which employees report each day.

Records for personnel who do not primarily report or work at a single establishment, such as traveling salesmen, technicians, engineers, etc., shall be maintained at the location from which they are paid or the base from which personnel operate to carry out their activities.

WORK ENVIRONMENT is comprised of the physical location, equipment, materials processed or used, and the kinds of operations performed in the course of an employee's work, wether on or off the employer's premisis.

APPENDIX M

Additional Web Resources

Online resources for the following topics that are available on the World Wide Web are listed in this appendix. (See also ANA's Safety and Health web page at www.nursingworld.org/dlwa/osh/.)

- Bloodborne pathogens (safer medical and needle devices)
- Ergonomics
- Formaldehyde
- Hazardous chemicals/gases
- Hazardous drugs
- Hazardous waste
- Hepatitis
- Human-immunodeficiency virus (HIV)
- Immunization safety
- Immunizations for health care workers
- Infection control/injury control
- Laser plume
- Latex allergies/sensitivities
- Methicillin resistant staphylococcus aureus (MRSA)
- Nitrous oxide
- Recordkeeping: OSHA compliance directives (CPLs)
- Respiratory protection
- Stress
- Tuberculosis
- Vancomycin resistant enterococcus (VRE)
- Workplace violence
- Miscellaneous sites

Bloodborne Pathogens (Safer Medical and Needle Devices)

- **Bloodborne Facts, fact sheets provided by OSHA entitled,**
  "Repeating Exposure Incidents"
  "Protect Yourself When Handling Sharps"
  "Hepatitis B Vaccination -Protection For You"
  " Personal Protective Equipment Cuts Risk, and Holding the line on contamination." Available: www.osha-slc.gov/OshDoc/data_BloodborneFacts/

■ Occupational Safety and Health Administration (OSHA). *Needlestick Injuries.* Includes final text of the 2000 amendments to the Bloodborne Pathogens Standard (29 CFR 1910.1030)
Available: www.osha-slc.gov/SLTC/needlestick/index.html

■ OSHA Compliance Directive. CPL 2-2.44D – *Enforcement Procedures of Occupational Exposure to Bloodborne Pathogens Standard.* Office of Health Compliance Assistance. U.S. Department of Labor. Occupational Safety and Health Administration. Washington, D.C. November 5, 1999.

Establishes policies and provides clarification to ensure uniform inspection procedures are followed when conducting inspections to enforce the Occupational Exposure to Bloodborne Pathogens Standard.
Available: www.Osha-slc.gov/OshDoc/Directive_data/CPL _2-2_44D.html

■ Food and Drug Administration (FDA) *Safety Alert: Needlestick and Other Risks from Hypodermic Needles on Secondary I.V. Administration Sets: Piggyback and Intermittent I.V.*
Available: www.osha-slc.gov/SLTC/needlestick/fdaletter.html

■ NIOSH Alert: *Preventing Needlestick Injuries in Health Care Settings* Publication No. 2000-108.Publication Date: 11/99
Available: www.cdc.gov/niosh/2000-108.html

■ NIOSH Guidelines for Selecting, Evaluating, and Using Sharps Disposal Containers. Publication No. 97-111, 1998. (To order, call 1-800-35NIOSH).
Available: www.cdc.gov/niosh/2000-108.html

■ California OSHA Sharps Injury Control Program. Include a listing of safer needle devices available on the market.
Available: www.ohb.org/sharps.htm

■ Training for the Development of Innovative Control Technologies (TDICT) Project. Includes needlestick device safety feature evaluation forms.
Available: www.tdict.org/criteria.html

■ ECRI: evaluation of needlestick devices.
Available: http://healthcare.ecri.org/site/whatsnew/press.releases/980723hdneedle.html

■ Exposure Prevention Information Network (EPINet) – Epidemiologic system for recording needlestick injuries developed by the Dr. Janine Jagger at the International Healthcare Worker Safety Center at the University of Virginia–Charlottesville.
Available: www.med.virginia.edu/~epinet

Ergonomics

■ Working Safely with Video Display Terminals. U.S. Department of Labor Occupational Safety and Health Administration. (OSHA 3092). 1997 (Revised)
Available: www. Osha-slc.gov/SLTC/ergonomics/index.html

■ **OSHA Ergonomic Standard**
Available: www.osha-slc.gov/ergonomics-standard/index.html

Formaldehyde

- CPL 2.2-52 – *Enforcement Procedure for Occupational Exposure to Formalde-hyde* (Information Date: 11/20/90)
  This instruction provides uniform inspection procedures and guidelines to be followed when conducting inspections and issuing citations for workers potentially exposed to formaldehyde.
  Available: www.osha-slc.gov/OshDoc/Directive_data/CPL_2- 2_52.html

Hazardous Chemicals/Gases

- *Managing Hazardous Materials Incidents, Volume I & II.* Emergency Medical, Services and Hospital Emergency Departments, U.S. Department of Human Services, Public Health Service, Agency for Toxic Substance and Disease Registry. Volume I and II
  Publication Date: 1/1/92
  http://aepo-xdv-www.epo.cdc.gov/wonder/prevguid/p0000018/0000018.htm
  http://aepo-xdv-www.epo.cdc.gov/wonder/prevguid/p0000019/0000019.htm

Hazardous Drugs

- *Controlling Occupational Exposure to Hazardous Drugs.* OSHA Technical Manual (TED 1-0.15A), Section VI, Chapter 2, (1999, January 20), 35 pages.
  Describes medical surveillance, handling, transporting, storing, and disposal of hazardous drugs. Appendix VI:2-1, contains common drugs considered hazardous. Appendix VI:2-2, contains aerosolized drugs considered to be hazardous.
  Available: www.osha-slc.gov/dts/osta/otm/otm_vi/otm_vi_2.html

- *Hospital Investigations: Health Hazards.* OSHA Technical Manual (TED 1-0.15A), Section IV, Chapter 1, (1999, January 20), 11 pages.
  Deals briefly with the hazards of anesthetic agents and antineoplastic drug exposures in the hospital setting.
  Available: www.osha-slc.gov/dts/osta/otm/otm_vi/otm_vi_1.html

Hazardous Waste

- Hazardous Waste and Emergency Response (OSHA 3114)

- OSHA Compliance Directive(s):

CPL 2-2.59A – Inspection Procedures for the Hazardous Waste Operations and Emergency Response Standard, 29 CFR 1910.120 and 1926.65, Paragraph (q): Emergency Response to Hazardous Substance Releases (Information Date: 4/24/98)

This instruction establishes policies an provides clarification to ensure uniform enforcement of paragraph (q) of the Hazardous Waste Operations and Emergency Response Standard (Hazwoper), 29 CFR 1910.120 and 1926.65, which covers emergency response operations for releases of, or substantial threats of releases of, hazardous substances without regard to the location of the hazard.

Hepatitis

- HESIS (Hazard Evaluation System and Information Service-Occupational Health Branch) Fact Sheet: Workplace Exposure to Hepatitis C. December 1998 Pp. 1-6. Available: www. Ohb.org/hcv.htm

- "Notice to Readers Recommendations for Follow-Up Health-Care Workers After Occupational Exposure to Hepatitis C Virus" *Morbidity and Mortality Weekly Report* 46(26), 603-606. Publication Date. 7/4/97. Available: www.Cdc.gov/epo/mmwr/preview/mmwrhtml/00048324.htm

- "Recommendations for Prevention and Control of Hepatitis C Virus (HCV) Infection and HCV-Related Chronic Disease" Morbidity and Mortality Weekly Report, 46(26), 603-606. Publication Date. 10/16/98 Available: www.cdc.gov/epo/mmwr/preview/mmwrhtml/00055154.htm

Human-Immunodeficiency Virus (HIV)

- *CDC/ATSDR Protocol for Handling Occupational Exposures to Human Immunodeficiency Virus (HIV)* (To order, send FAX to 404-639-3883). Publication Date: 11/10/92
  Available: http://aepo-xdv-www.epo.cdc.gov/wonder/prevguid/p0000085/p0000085.htm

- "First-Line Drugs for HIV Postexposure Prophylaxis (PEP)." (Appendix). Morbidity and Mortality Weekly Report, 47(RR-7);29-30. May 15, 1998. Available: www.cdc.gov/epo/mmwr/preview/mmwrhtml/00052801.htm

- "Public Health Service Guidelines for the Management of Health-Care Worker Exposures to HIV and Recommendations for Postexposure Prophylaxis." CDC *MMWR Recommendations and Reports.* May 15, 1998, 47 (RR-7); 1-28.
  Available: www.cdc.gov/epo/Mmwr/preview/mmwrhtml/00052722.htm

- "Reported Cases of AIDS and HIV Infection In Health Care Workers." Division of HIV/AIDS Prevention. Centers for Disease Control and Prevention. May 13,1999 ; pp 1-2.
  Available: www.cdc.gov/hiv/hivinfo/vfax/260230.htm

Immunization Safety

- Food and Drug Administration (FDA)
  Available: www.fda.gov/fdac/features/095_vacc.html
  www.fda.gov/cber/vaers/vaers.htm

  The first site features information about how the FDA ensures vaccine safety. The second site has information on the Vaccine Adverse Event Reporting System (VAERS), a cooperative program for vaccine safety of the FDA and the CDC.

- Immunization of Health Care Workers: Recommendations of the Advisory Committee on Immunization Practices (ACIP) and the Hospital Infection Control Practices Advisory Committee (HICPAC). Publication Date: 12/26/1997. (Provides recommendations for Hepatitis B).

- World Health Organization (WHO).

  Features a Vaccine Safety home page which offers links to vaccine safety related information.
  Available: www.who.int/vaccines-diseases/

Immunizations for Health Care Workers

- Centers for Disease Control and Prevention (CDC).

  The National Immunization Program (NIP) of the CDC features information on vaccine safety.
  Available: www. Cdc.gov/nip/vacsafe

- Protections against Viral Hepatitis Recommendations of the Immunization Practices Advisory Committee (ACIP). MMWR 39(RR-2). February 9,1990. Centers for Disease Control
  Available: www.cdc.gov/mmwr/preview/mmwrhtml/00041917.htm

Infection Control/Injury Control

- Bolyard, E. A. Tablan, O.C. Williams, W.W., Pearson, M.L., Shapiro, C.N., Deitchman, S.D. and The Hospital Infection Control Practices Advisory Committee. 1998. *Guideline for Infection Control in Health Care Personnel. Centers for Disease Control and Prevention.*
  Available: www.cdc.gov/ncidod/hip/guide/infectcontrol98.pdf

  [Published simultaneously in *American Journal of Infection Control* (1998;26:289-354) and *Infection Control and Hospital Epidemiology* (1998;19:407-63).]

- *CDC Prevention Guidelines Database*

  A compilation of all of the official guidelines and recommendations published by the CDC for the prevention of diseases, disabilities, and injuries.
  Available: http://aepo-xdv-www.epo.cdc.gov/wonder/prevguid/prevguid.htm

- *Morbidity and Mortality Weekly Report* (MMWR).

  Contains comprehensive information on policy statements for prevention and treatment that are within the CDC's scope of responsibility.
  Available: www2.cdc.gov/mmwr/mmwr.html

Laser Plume

- *Hospital Investigations: Health Hazards.* OSHA Technical Manual (TED-0.15A), Section VI-Chapter 1. Describes lasers as a potential hazard in the hospital environment and identifies areas to investigate. January 20, 1999.
  Available: www.osha-slc.gov/SLTC/laserhazards/index.html

- NIOSH Hazard Controls (HC11) – *Control of Smoke from Laser/Electric Surgical Procedures.* Publication No. 96-128.
  Available: Www.cdc.gov/niosh/hc11.html

Latex Allergies/Sensitivities

- *Latex Allergy.* NIOSH Facts. June 1997.
  Available: www.cdc.gov/niosh/latexfs.html

- *Preventing Allergic Reactions to Rubber Latex in the Workplace.* NIOSH Alert. Publication No. 97-135. June 1, 1997. Describes and defines types of latex

reactions occurring in people using or working with latex products. It also describes how the allergy occurs.
Available: www.osha-slc.gov/SLTC/latexallergy/index.html

■ *OSHA Technical Information Bulletin- Potential for Allergy to Natural Rubber Latex Gloves and Other Natural Rubber Products.* April 12,1999. OSHA
Available: www.osha-slc.gov/html/hotfoias/tib/TIB19990412.html

■ American College of Allergy, Asthma, and Immunology. Latex Allergy home page includes Guidelines for the Management of Latex Allergy and Safe Latex Use in Health Care Facilities.
http://allergy.mch.edu/physicians/ltxhome.html

■ Latex Allergy links
www.netcom.com/~nam1latex_allergy.html

Methicillin Resistant Staphylococcus Aureus (MRSA)

■ *Methicillin Resistant Staphylococcus Aureus: Facts for Health Care Workers. 1999.* Available: www.cdc.gov/ncidod/hip/aresist/mrsahcw.htm

Nitrous Oxide

■ NIOSH Hazard Controls (HC29) – Control of Nitrous Oxide During Cryosurgery. Publication No. 99-105. Publication Date: 1/99. U.S. Department of Health and Human Services. NIOSH.
Available: www.cdc.gov/niosh/hc29.html

■ *NIOSH Alert: Controlling Exposures to Nitrous Oxide During Anesthetic Administration. Publication.* No. 94-100. Publication Date: 1994. U.S. Department of Health and Human Services. NIOSH.
Available: www.cdc.gov/niosh/noxidalr.html

Recordkeeping: OSHA Compliance Directives (CPLs)

■ CPL 2-2.46 – 29 CFR 1913. 10(b) (6), *Authorization and Procedures for Reviewing Specific Medical Records to Verify Compliance with 29 CFR 1904.* Information Date: 1/5/89.

This instruction authorizes appropriately qualified OSHA personnel to conduct reviews of the medical records where there is a need to gain access to verify compliance with 29 CFR 1904 recordkeeping requirements.
Available: www.osha-slc.gov/OshDoc/Directive_data/CPL_2-2_33.html

■ CPL 2-2.33 – Standard Number: 1913.10; 1910.20 Subject: 29 CFR 1913.10, *Rules of Agency Practice and Procedure Concerning OSHA Access to Employee Medical Records: Procedures Governing Enforcement Activities.* Information Date: 2/8/1982.

This instruction provides guidance for implementing the rules of agency practice and procedure concerning OSHA access to employee medical records.
Available: www.osha.slc.gov/OshDoc/Directive_data/CPL_2-2_33.html

■ CPL 2-2.30 – 29 CFR 1913.10(b)(6), *Authorization of Review of Medical Opinions.* Information *Date*1/14/80.

This instruction authorizes appropriately qualities OSHA personnel to conduct reviews of medical opinions mandated by specific occupational safety and health standards where there is a need to gain access for enforcement purposes.
Available: www.osha-slc.gov/OshDoc/Directive_data/CPL_2-2_30.html

Respiratory Protection

OSHA Compliance Directives:

■ CPL 2-0.120 – Inspection Procedures for the Respiratory Protection Standard. Information Date: 9/25/98.

This instruction establishes agency interpretations and enforcement policies, and provides instructions to ensure uniform enforcement of the Respiratory Protection Standard, 29 CFR 1910.134.
Available: www.osha-slc.gov/OshDoc/Directive_data/CPL_2-0_120.html

Safer Medical/Needle Devices

(See Bloodborne Pathogens section.)

Stress

■ NIOSH, *Stress at Work*
www.cdc.gov/niosh/99-101pd.html

Tuberculosis

■ *Core Curriculum on Tuberculosis: What the Clinician Should Know.* 4th ed. 2000. U.S. Department of Health and Human Services. Centers for Disease Control and Prevention.
Available: www.cdc.gov/nchstp/tb/pubs/corecurr/

■ *OSHA Fact Sheet: Enforcement Policy on Tuberculosis #93-43.* January 1, 1993.
Available: www.osha-slc.gov/OshDoc/Fact_data/FSNo93-43.html

■ Guidelines for Preventing the Transmission of Mycobacterium Tuberculosis in Health-Care Facilities. October 28, 1994. *Morbidity and Mortality Weekly Report,* 43(RR-13); 1-132. U.S. Department of Health and Human Services. Centers for Disease Control and Prevention.
Available: http://aepo-xdv-www.cdc.gov/wonder/prevguid/m0035909/m0035909.htm

■ *Guidelines for the Prevention of Tuberculosis in Health Care Facilities in Resource-limited Settings.* World Health Organizations. 1999.
Available: www.who.int/gtb/publications/healthcare/index.htm

■ Prevention and Control of Tuberculosis in Facilities Providing Long-Term Care to the Elderly Recommendations of the Advisory Committee for Elimination of Tuberculosis. *Morbidity and Mortality Weekly Report,* 39(RR-10); 7-20. Publication Date: 7/13/90
Available: http://aepo-xdv-www.epo.cdc.gov/wonder/prevguid/pOO00185/pOO00185.htm

■ *Protect Yourself Against Tuberculosis: A Respiratory Protection Guide for Health Care Workers.* Publication No. 96-102. Publication Date: 12/95.
Available: www.cdc.gov/niosh/tb.html

■ *The Role of BCG Vaccine in Prevention and Control of Tuberculosis in the United States.* CDC MMWR 45(RR-4). Publication Date: April 26,1996.
Available: www.cdc.gov/nchstp/tb/Pubs/Mmwr/rr4504.pdf

■ *Screening for Tuberculosis and Tuberculosis Infection in High Risk Populations: Recommendations of the Advisory Council for the Elimination of Tuberculosis.* CDC MMWR 44(RR-11)18–34. Publication Date: September 8, 1995.
Available: http://wonder.cdc.gov/wonder/prevguid/m0038873/m0038873.asp

■ *Recommendations of the Advisory Council for the Elimination of Tuberculosis,* 44(RR- 11), 18-34. September 8, 1995.
Available: www.cdc.gov/epo/mmwr/preview/mmwrhtml/00038873.htm

■ TB: Respiratory Protection Program in Health Care Facilities - Administrator's Guide Publication No. 99-143.Publication Date: 9/99.
Available: www.cdc.gov/niosh/99-143

■ Tuberculosis Control Laws - United States: Recommendations of the Advisory Council for the Elimination of Tuberculosis. *Morbidity and Mortality Weekly Report* 42(RR-15). Publication Date: 11/12/93
Available: www.cdc.gov/epo/mmwr/preview/mmwrhtml/00030715.htm

■ The Use of Preventive Therapy for Tuberculosis Infection in the United States: Recommendations of the Advisory Committee for Elimination of Tuberculosis. *Morbidity and Mortality Weekly Report* 39(RR-8); 9-12. Publication Date: 5/15/90
Available: http://aepo-xdv-www.epo.cdc.gov/wonder/prevguid/m0001643/0001643.htm

■ OSHA Compliance Directive (CPL)

CPL 2.106 – Enforcement Procedures and Scheduling for Occupational Exposure to Tuberculosis. Information Date: 2/9/1996.

Vancomycin Resistant Enterococcus (VRE)

Recommendations for Preventing the Spread of Vancomycin Resistance. Recommendations of the Hospital Infection Control Practices Advisory Committee (HICPAC). September 22, 1995. *Morbidity and Mortality Weekly Report,* 44(RR12), pp 1-l-3.
Available: http://aepo-xdv-www.epo.cdc.gov/wonder/prevguid/m0039349/m0039349.htm

■ Hospital Infections Program. National Center for Disease and Prevention. 1999.
Available: www.cdc.gov/ncidod/hip/aresist/vre.htm

Workplace Violence

■ *NIOSH Facts: Violence in the Workplace.* June 1997
Available: www.cdc.gov/niosh/violfs.html

- *OSHA Guidelines for Preventing Workplace Violence for Healthcare and Social Service Workers.*
  Available: www.osha-slc.gov/SLTC/workplaceviolence/guideline.html

Miscellaneous Sites

- National Institute for Occupational Safety and Health (NIOSH). *Guidelines for Protecting the Safety and Health of Health Care Workers.*
  Available: www.cdc.gov/niosh/pdfs/88-119.pdf

- U.S. Department of Labor, Occupational Safety and Health Administration. *Worker Rights Under the Occupational Safety and Health Act of 1970.*
  Available: www.odhs.gov/as/opa/worker/rights.html

- U.S. Department of Labor, Occupational Safety and Health Administration. *Employer Responsibility.*
  Available: www.osh.gov/as/opa/worker/employer-responsibility.html

- U.S. Department of Labor, Occupational Safety and Health Administration. *Nursing Home Electronic Compliance Assistance Tool (eCAT). A Virtual Nursing Home Walk-through for Health and Safety.*
  Available: www.osha-slc.gov/SLTC/nursinghome_ecat/index.html

- American College of Occupational and Environmental Medicine (ACOEM) *Guidelines for Employee Health Services in Health Care Facilities.*
  Available: www.occenvmed.net

- Sustainable Hospitals Project (SHP)

  The Sustainable Hospitals Project at the University of Massachusetts–Lowell has a web-based clearinghouse for selecting products and work practices that eliminate or reduce occupational and environmental hazards, maintain quality patient care, and contain costs. Information about latex-free medical gloves, safer needle devices, alternatives to polyvinyl chloride products (PVC), and mercury-free products are included at this site.
  Available: www.sustainablehospitals.org

- Health Care Without Harm (HCWH)
  Available: www.noharm.org

APPENDIX N

OSHA's New Recordkeeping Rule: OSHA 300 Log

On January 19, 2001 OSHA issued a revised rule changing the requirements employers must follow for recording injuries and illnesses in the workplace. The new recordkeeping rule, a revision of 29 CFR Part 1904, becomes effective on January 1, 2002.

This appendix describes the new rule and the new form (OSHA 300 Log) and notes what has changed from the previous rule and the use of the old form (OSHA 200 Log). At the end of this appendix, the two forms are compared in Figure N-1; the OSHA 300 Log is reproduced on pages 102 and 103.

Who Is Covered By The Revised Rule?
[1904.1 and 1904.2]

All employers covered by OSHA who have more than 10 employees in the entire company are required to keep records of injuries and illnesses. Employers in certain low hazard industries involving retail, service, finance, insurance, or the real estate industry are exempt from these recordkeeping requirements.

What Changed?

There were some changes made to the list of "low hazard" industries that are to be exempt from OSHA's new recordkeeping requirements. For example, industrial laundries are no longer considered "low hazard" and will now be required to keep OSHA 300 Logs. On the other hand, offices and clinics of medical doctors and dentists will no longer be required to keep injury and illness logs under the revised rule.

What Injuries/Illnesses Must The Employer Record?
[1904.4 - 1904.12]

Employers must record all new cases of work-related fatalities, injuries, and illnesses if they involve:

- Death
- Days away from work
- Restricted work or transfer to another job
- Medical treatment beyond first aid
- Loss of consciousness
- A significant injury or illness diagnosed by a physician or other licensed health care professional

What Changed?

The old rule required *all* occupational illnesses to be recorded. The new rule dropped that requirement, but added a new category of injuries/illnesses for employers to record, called "significant injury or illness diagnosed by a physician or other licensed health care professional." This includes such injuries/illnesses as work-related cancer, chronic irreversible diseases such as silicosis, a fractured or cracked bone and a punctured eardrum.

The new rule made some changes in the definition of "first aid" cases, allowing, for example, injuries that are treated with hot or cold compresses on more than one occasion to be considered "first aid" cases and therefore not required to be recorded on the OSHA 300 Log.

New criteria were added to the revised rule for recording needlestick and sharps injury cases where objects are contaminated with another person's blood or other potentially infectious material; tuberculosis cases; occupational hearing loss cases; medical removal cases under OSHA standards; and work-related musculoskeletal disorders.

The new rule also identified certain injuries and illnesses that, while they may occur at work, do not have to be recorded on the OSHA 300 Log. These include situations such as an injury that occurs as a result of an employee choking on a sandwich while at work, an injury/illness resulting from voluntary participation in a wellness program or recreational activity, and an injury caused by a motor vehicle accident in a company parking lot while the employee is commuting to or from work.

The new rule also clarified what is deemed recordable and non-recordable regarding injuries and illnesses that occur to workers when they are on work-related travel assignments.

New Forms Used For Recording Injuries And Illnesses [1904.29]

New forms will be used to record work-related injuries and illnesses. Employers will use:

- The OSHA 300 Log of Work-Related Injuries and Illnesses to record all injuries and illnesses. It will replace the old OSHA 200 Log. (Seethe end of this appendix for a copy of the new OSHA 300 log).

- Form 300-A is the Summary of Work-Related Injuries and Illnesses, which is to be posted in the workplace annually.

- Form 301 is called the Injury and Illness Incident Report, which is used to record information on how each injury or illness case occurred. It replaces the old Form 101, the Supplementary Record of Occupational Injuries and Illnesses.

Each recordable injury or illness case must be recorded on the OSHA 300 Log and the 301 Incident Report within seven (7) calendar days after the employer receives notice that the injury or illness occurred.

What Changed?

The new OSHA Log 300 no longer asks for the department in which an employee is regularly employed, but instead asks where the event (injury/illness) occurred.

Instead of dividing the form between "injuries" and "illnesses," as the old OSHA 200 Log does, the OSHA 300 Log requires employers to check one of seven boxes to categorize the injury/illness. Those seven categories are:

■ Injury

■ Musculoskeletal disorder (this would include everything from carpal tunnel syndrome to low back pain)

■ Skin disorder

■ Respiratory condition

■ Poisoning

■ Hearing loss

■ All other illnesses

There are still spaces to record days of job transfer or work restriction, as well as days away from work. The term "lost workday", which was used on the OSHA 200 Log, has been eliminated

Summary Form 300-A makes summary workplace injury/illness information (to be posted annually) easier to understand and evaluate than the previous summary form.

Issues of Privacy and Recording Injuries and Illnesses [1904.29]

The new rule prohibits the employer from entering an employee's name on the OSHA 300 Log to protect the privacy of the injured or ill worker in cases where the injury or illness occurred to an intimate body part or the reproductive system; sexual assaults; mental illnesses; HIV infection, hepatitis, or tuberculosis; and needlestick injuries and cuts from sharps where the objects are contaminated with another person's blood. In these privacy concern cases, a separate confidential list of employee names must be kept. Employers also have the right to use discretion in describing the sensitive nature of the injury where the worker's identity would be known.

The incident still will be recorded but without identifying the employee's name.

What Changed?

The rules regarding "privacy concern cases" are entirely new, and did not exist under the old rule.

Which Employees Are Covered By The Recording Requirements? [1904.31]

The employer is required to record on the OSHA 300 Log the recordable injuries and illnesses for all employees on its payroll, including hourly, salaried, executive, part-time, seasonal, or migrant workers. The employer must also record injuries and illnesses that occur to workers who are *not* on the employers payroll if the employer supervises these workers on a *day-to-day* basis.

What Changed?

Employers will now be required to record injuries and illnesses that affect workers that they supervise on a day-to-day basis, including employees of temporary help services, employee leasing services, personnel supply services, and contractors.

The Annual Summary [1904.32]

At the end of each calendar year, the 300-A Summary form of the total recordable injuries and illnesses for that year must be completed and certified by a company executive as correct and complete. The annual summary must be posted in the workplace where notices to workers are usually posted. The summary of the previous year's recordable injuries and illnesses is required to be posted for three months beginning on February 1 until April 30.

What Changed?

Employers will be required to post the annual summary (now called Form 300 A) for 3 months (February 1 – April 30) instead of only one month (the month of February).

Keeping The Injury and Illness Records [1904.33]

The employer must save the OSHA 300 Log, the Form 300-A Annual Summary, any privacy case list, and the Form 301 Incident Report forms for five (5) years. The stored Form 300 Logs must be updated by the employer to include any newly discovered recordable injuries or illnesses.

What Changed?

There were no changes in this requirement.

Employees Must Be Involved [1904.35]

Under the new rules, employers are required to inform workers how they are to report injuries or illnesses and set up a way to receive these reports promptly. The employer must also provide workers, former workers, their personal representatives, and their authorized employee representative (union representative) with access to injury and illness records, including a copy of the OSHA 300 Logs by the end of the next business day. The names of employees must be left on the OSHA 300 Log unless they are "privacy concern cases."

Employees, former employees, or personal representatives must be given a copy of a requested Form 301 Incident Report by the end of the next business day. When an authorized employee representative (union representative) asks for a copy of the Form 301 Incident Report, the employer is required to give copies of the part of the form that contains information about the case, with all personal information removed, within 7 calendar days.

Employers must provide copies of the OSHA 300 Logs and Form 301 Incident Report free of charge the first time they are requested.

What Changed?

Time limits for employers to provide recordkeeping information to workers, union representatives and others have been established.

Employees, former employees and personal representatives will now have legal rights to obtain the more detailed information about their own injuries/illnesses, recorded on the OSHA Form 301 Incident Report Form. Union representatives will have access to a portion of OSHA Form 301, specifically the "Information About the Case" section with all personal identifiers removed.

The new OSHA 300 Log allows employers to withhold the names, and in some situations the details, of "privacy concern cases." These are cases involving such incidents and illnesses as sexual assault, HIV, and tuberculosis.

FIGURE N-1. COMPARISON BETWEEN OSHA 200 AND OSHA 300 LOGS.

Category Heading	OSHA 200 Log Column	OSHA 300 Log Column
Case number	A	same (A)
Employee's name	C	B (see new privacy language: name will not be recorded for certain injuries/illnesses)
Job title	D	C
Date of injury or		
Onset of illness	B	D
Department of employee	E	No longer recorded; see the column, Where the event occurred
Where the event occurred	not applicable	E (new)
Description of injury or illness	F	same (F)
Date of death (check if death from injury or illness) occurred	1 & 8: date of death	G: Check if death
Check if days lost from work	2–3 (injury), 9–10 (illness)	H
Check if restricted duty/light duty	2 (due to injury), 9 (due to illness)	I
Number of days on restricted duty	5, 12	K
Number of days away from work	4, 11	L
Check if injury	2, 6	M-1
Injury or illness without lost or restricted work days	6 (injury); 13 (illness)	J
Check type of illness:		
▪ Musculoskeletal disorder	7 (f)	M-2
▪ Skin disorder	7 (a)	M-3
▪ Respiratory condition	7 (b & c)	M-4 combined dust and toxic causes of respiratory condition (may check either or both M-3 and M-4 for latex allergy)
▪ Poisoning	7 (d)	M-5
▪ Hearing loss	none (new)	M-6
▪ All other illnesses	7 (g)	M-7
▪ Disorder due to physical agents	7(e)	None (discontinued category)

OSHA's Form 300

Log of Work-Related Injuries and Illnesses

You must record information about every work-related death and about every work-related injury or illness that involves loss of consciousness, restricted work activity or job transfer, days away from work, or medical treatment beyond first aid. You must also record significant work-related injuries and illnesses that are diagnosed by a physician or licensed health care professional. You must also record work-related injuries and illnesses that meet any of the specific recording criteria listed in 29 CFR Part 1904.8 through 1904.12. Feel free to use two lines for a single case if you need to. You must complete an Injury and Illness Incident Report (OSHA Form 301) or equivalent form for each injury or illness recorded on this form. If you're not sure whether a case is recordable, call your local OSHA office for help.

Attention: This form contains information relating to employee health and must be used in a manner that protects the confidentiality of employees to the extent possible while the information is being used for occupational safety and health purposes.

Year 20____

U.S. Department of Labor
Occupational Safety and Health Administration

Form approved OMB no. 1218-0176

Establishment name _____

City _____ State _____

Identify the person

(A) Case no.	(B) Employee's name	(C) Job title (e.g., Welder)

Describe the case

(D) Date of injury or onset of illness	(E) Where the event occurred (e.g., Loading dock north end)	(F) Describe injury or illness, parts of body affected, and object/substance that directly injured or made person ill (e.g., Second degree burns on right forearm from acetylene torch)
___/___ month/day		

Classify the case

Using these four categories, check ONLY the most serious result for each case:

(G) Death	(H) Days away from work	(I) Remained at work — Job transfer or restriction	(J) Remained at work — Other recordable cases
☐	☐	☐	☐

Enter the number of days the injured or ill worker was:

(K) On job transfer or restriction	(L) Away from work
____ days	____ days

Check the "injury" column or choose one type of illness:

(M) (1) Injury	(2) Skin disorder	(3) Respiratory condition	(4) Poisoning	(5) Hearing loss	(6) All other illnesses
☐	☐	☐	☐	☐	☐

Page totals ▶

| | | | | | ____ | ____ | (1) | (2) | (3) | (4) | (5) | (6) |

Be sure to transfer these totals to the Summary page (Form 300A) before you post it.

Injury | Skin disorder | Respiratory condition | Poisoning | Hearing loss | All other illnesses
(1) (2) (3) (4) (5) (6) (7)

Page ____ of ____

Public reporting burden for this collection of information is estimated to average 14 minutes per response, including time to review the instructions, search and gather the data needed, and complete and review the collection of information. Persons are not required to respond to the collection of information unless it displays a currently valid OMB control number. If you have any comments about these estimates or any other aspects of this data collection, contact: US Department of Labor, OSHA Office of Statistics, Room N-3644, 200 Constitution Avenue, NW, Washington, DC 20210. Do not send the completed forms to this office.

OSHA's Form 300A

Summary of Work-Related Injuries and Illnesses

All establishments covered by Part 1904 must complete this Summary page, even if no work-related injuries or illnesses occurred during the year. Remember to review the Log to verify that the entries are complete and accurate before completing this summary.

Using the Log, count the individual entries you made for each category. Then write the totals below, making sure you've added the entries from every page of the Log. If you had no cases, write "0."

Employees, former employees, and their representatives have the right to review the OSHA Form 300 in its entirety. They also have limited access to the OSHA Form 301 or its equivalent. See 29 CFR Part 1904.35, in OSHA's recordkeeping rule, for further details on the access provisions for these forms.

Number of Cases

Total number of deaths	Total number of cases with days away from work	Total number of cases with job transfer or restriction	Total number of other recordable cases
___ (G)	___ (H)	___ (I)	___ (J)

Number of Days

Total number of days of job transfer or restriction	Total number of days away from work
___ (K)	___ (L)

Injury and Illness Types

Total number of . . .
(M)

(1) Injuries ___
(2) Musculoskeletal disorders ___
(3) Skin disorders ___
(4) Respiratory conditions ___
(5) Poisonings ___
(6) Hearing loss cases ___
(7) All other illnesses ___

Establishment information

Your establishment name ___

Street ___

City ___ State ___ ZIP ___

Industry description (e.g., Manufacture of motor truck trailers) ___

Standard Industrial Classification (SIC), if known (e.g., SIC 3715) ___ — ___ — ___ —

Employment information (If you don't have these figures, see the Worksheet on the back of this page to estimate.)

Annual average number of employees ___

Total hours worked by all employees last year ___

Sign here

Knowingly falsifying this document may result in a fine.

I certify that I have examined this document and that to the best of my knowledge the entries are true, accurate, and complete.

Company executive ___ Title ___

(___) ___ - ___ ___/___/___
Phone   Date

Post this Summary page from February 1 to April 30 of the year following the year covered by the form.

Public reporting burden for this collection of information is estimated to average 50 minutes per response, including time to review the instructions, search and gather the data needed, and complete and review the collection of information. Persons are not required to respond to the collection of information unless it displays a currently valid OMB control number. If you have any comments about these estimates or any other aspects of this data collection, contact: US Department of Labor, OSHA Office of Statistics, Room N-3644, 200 Constitution Avenue, NW, Washington, DC 20210. Do not send the completed forms to this office.